Enduring
Shame

Enduring
Shame

A Recent History of
Unwed Pregnancy
and Righteous
Reproduction

Heather Brook Adams

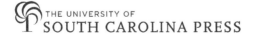
THE UNIVERSITY OF
SOUTH CAROLINA PRESS

© 2022 University of South Carolina

Published by the University of South Carolina Press
Columbia, South Carolina 29208

www.uscpress.com

Manufactured in the United States of America

31 30 29 28 27 26 25 24 23 22
10 9 8 7 6 5 4 3 2 1

Library of Congress Cataloging-in-Publication Data
can be found at http://catalog.loc.gov/.

ISBN: 978-1-64336-293-9 (hardcover)
ISBN: 978-1-64336-294-6 (paperback)
ISBN: 978-1-64336-295-3 (ebook)

In loving memory of Ludmilla,
and the innumerable women like her

Contents

Illustrations

Acknowledgments

Writing a book across years, locations, and political contexts has been a complex affair—a vacillation between "just send it out" and "rethink and reshape." Now I realize that a book is a phenomenon that can and should assume the space it needs. Foundational research for this project was possible because of support from Pennsylvania State University, including the Center for Democratic Deliberation. A University of North Carolina Greensboro (UNCG) New Faculty Award and a UNCG Marc Friedlaender Faculty Excellence Award in English enabled significant research, interviews, and development. Essential work at the University of Minnesota Social Welfare History Archive was possible thanks to a Clarke Chambers Travel Fellowship and the generous assistance of archivists Linnea Anderson and David Klassen.

Chapter 1 includes material from my article "Rhetorics of Unwed Motherhood and Shame" in *Women's Studies in Communication* 40, no.1 (2017) copyright © Organization for Research on Women and Communication, reprinted by permission of Taylor & Francis Ltd, www.tandfonline.com, on behalf of Organization for Research on Women and Communication. A portion of chapter 3 was drawn from my essay "The Feminist Work of Unsticking Shame: Affective Realignment in the 1973 Edition of Our Bodies, Ourselves," published in *Peitho* 21, no. 3 (2019). A special thank you to Megan J. Smith for permitting me to share her artwork in this book.

I owe a debt of gratitude to many people, starting with Cristian Núñez, "research assistant" extraordinaire and life partner. For innumerable reasons, without you this project would not be.

Cheryl Glenn's brilliance is the inspiration for and the foundation of this book. Her labor to help me trust my mind and voice is as generous a gift as I could imagine. Cheryl, you are, simply, unparalleled in grace, magnanimity, and verve. My appreciation, dear friend, will never feel sufficient.

Special thanks to the mothers who were willing to meet with me, open their homes and lives to me, and to share a most sacred part of their experience. I appreciate your patience and hope I have honored your wisdom on these pages.

Aurora Bell, editor of the highest caliber, and two anonymous and generous readers enabled me to deepen the project in significant ways. Our field is fortunate for University of South Carolina Press Director Richard Brown's interest and ethical approach to supporting emerging writers.

Mari Boor Tonn first encouraged me to pursue this research. Since then, I have benefitted from the wisdom and encouragement of many: Jack Selzer, Lindal Buchanan, Charlotte Hogg, David Gold, J. Michael Hogan, Hester Blum, Jason Barrett-Fox, Michael Faris, Ersula Ore, Bonnie Sierlecki, Emily Winderman, Sarah Singer, David Green, Mark Hlavacik, Matt Biddle, John Belk, Laura Brown, Sarah Summers, Stacey Sheriff, Judy Holiday, Heather Blaine Vorhees, Jervette Ward, Timothy Barney, Ben Krueger, Elizabeth Gardner, and Jenna Vinson. Michelle Smith remains my two-steps ahead mentor, for which I am grateful. Sarah Hallenbeck unselfishly shared with me time and insight and has been a tremendous academic role model. Jessica Enoch's, Jordynn Jack's, and Wendy Sharer's influences are suffused throughout this book. Jess, in our very first conversation we spoke of your recently published monograph; you assured me that "Someday, you'll have one of those too." Those words have stuck with me and buoyed me through moments of doubt.

Gratitude to UNCG colleagues—Jennifer Feather, Jennifer Keith, Amy Vines, Karen Kilcup, Nancy Myers, Steve Yarbrough, Scott Romine, María Sánchez, Karen Weyler, Christian Moraru, and Anne Wallace—who have cared for me and this project in various and essential ways. I extend appreciation to UNCG College of Arts and Sciences Dean John Kiss for his earnest enthusiasm for my work as a member of the junior faculty in the Department of English. Friends in Agraphia and Write-on-Site have shared accountability and the conviviality of writing in community. To Anne Parsons, Paul Silvia, Cybelle McFadden, and Lisa Tolbert: special thanks for your sustained and timely support and yes, I met my writing goals for the week.

Ronald Spatz imagines writers' vast and vibrant possibilities, plus he gives the best pep talks. Ron, your patience, fortitude, and friendship mean the world to me. Jennifer Mallette, accountability partner-turned-cherished friend, thank you for keeping me on track in all the ways. Risa Applegarth, you honor me with curiosity, expertly posed queries, generative ideas, problem-solving sessions, and stunning ingenuity. May we write together for years to come.

Care and community shape a writer and her writing. Margaret Hoff and Jamey Bradbury motivate me, lift me with laughter, and are two of the best friends and writers I know. Unending love to Alyse Knorr, Kate Partridge, Jackie Cason, Trish Jenkins, Ray Ball, Emily Madsen, Camilla Madden, Sarah Dalrymple Foster, Patty Balboni, Gertrude Beal, MJ Knight, and Sarah Estow. Each of you have, in some way, helped me achieve this goal.

To my mother, Phyllis Adams, boundless gratitude for loving me enough to help me pursue my passion. Your sacrifices have been many, and I love you. Quiero agradecer a mis suegros, Dassy y Eduardo, por mostrarme y brindarme, a mí, su "hijita," la belleza del amor incondicional. Cris, everlasting appreciation for listening as I "talked it out" and responding with your whole mind and soul. Your intellectual companionship has been the bedrock of my discernment. Thank you for always making me coffee and for sharing this grand adventure with me. Last but in no way least, I hope this book honors the unforgettable spirit and life of my father, Arden Adams, whose lessons and love continue to carry me onward.

Introduction

Sex, Shame, and Rhetoric

I.

t is 1954. "Louise,"[1] 22 years old, pregnant, and unmarried, enters the Roselia Foundling and Maternity Asylum in Pittsburgh, Pennsylvania. Like thousands of other women in her situation, Louise is gripped with fear and shame because of her unwed pregnancy. Going to the maternity home, which is four hours away from her rural Pennsylvania hometown, will allow Louise to hide, anonymously, during her pregnancy and to surrender her child for adoption. About twenty-five other unwed mothers also hide in the home. Together, the women play solitaire, keep up with daily chores, and pass the time until they give birth. Louise will return to her hometown after she delivers a child she never sees again. Despite her family's effort to keep her pregnancy a secret, people know and talk. Louise meets the man she will eventually marry, and his friends try to talk him out of dating "that kind of girl." He refuses to listen. Louise and her husband hold the secret of her past even now, as a couple in their 80s. I talk to them on a day when their daughter is not likely to stop by the house.

II.

It is 2017. Journalist, researcher, and Yale Law School lecturer Emily Bazelon discusses the idea of "coming forward" to identify moments of sexual misconduct amid a burgeoning #MeToo movement on the podcast she cohosts, "Political Gabfest." She shares her personal experience of interacting with magazine editor Leon Wieseltier.

> The one time I met him, I thought he was a total, lecherous jerk. He probably doesn't even remember that. I wasn't working for him, but it is, like, a memory I definitely have. So in this discussion of "why don't people come forward earlier?" and "when everyone knows this about someone, why does it continue?" In that moment there's so much shame. And you

blame yourself and you feel weird about it. I can't even remember whether I went home and told my husband like the weird, yucky thing that I experienced at dinner with Leon Wieseltier 'cause I was, like, 28. And it made me feel worried that I had done something to bring it on, the environment it happened in made me feel like, you know, that there was something probably wrong with me—um, or just that he had power and I didn't.

Continuing to reflect upon the act of breaking the silence surrounding sexual misconduct, Bazelon adds:

It's only obvious in retrospect, right? It's like once the momentum starts and Gwyneth Paltrow is on the front page of the *New York Times* making these sober accusations we see that as heroic and honorable. And then we start pointing fingers at everyone—all the men around, all the other women around—some of whom were part of this or enabled it. And it seems so obvious, like, who is good and who is bad and who's up and who's down but before it breaks, like, it's not the *least bit* clear that it is going to play out that way. (Bazelon, Dickerson, and Plotz 2017)

———•———

What use comes from putting these two moments, sixty-three years apart, side by side? Initially, the disparity between women's limited sexual freedoms of the 1950s and the collective resistance against sexual violence represented by the events of 2017 seems great—an illustration of the radically different life experiences of women across two centuries in relation to their sexual identities, capabilities, and constraints. I have chosen these seemingly incongruous moments in time, however, to serve as a representative frame for this book, which identifies how shame, as emotion and rhetorical resource, functions as an ongoing, powerful, and misunderstood aspect of women's sexual and reproductive experiences in the United States since the mid twentieth century. Attention to this rhetorical gendered history can deepen any number of investigations into wider sites of injustice related to reproducing people—people who identify as women or who can or try to reproduce. Too often public narratives of women's sexual and reproductive lives represent a story of steady progress that is threatened by backlash politics or efforts to roll back reproductive gains. That common story is both true and not true, a simplified version of gendered power that masks the fragility of women's ability to manage their own fertility and enjoy sovereignty over their sexual lives. Without a more complete story, this notion of progress remains dangerously deficient. A fuller understanding would consider changes that have made headlines alongside stories that remain silenced or have been purposefully ignored. A more robust story would better account for the lived experiences of various people (not just affluent white reproducing women). A more comprehensive telling of recent reproductive history (i.e., from the 1950s forward) would explore the feelings and perceptions of the women who lived through moments of change. This book offers one such story—fuller, if surely still incomplete.

Public stories of the reproductive changes that have taken place within the lifetime of many people alive today circulate widely but are perfunctory. Their partiality ultimately weakens all women's ability to know the possibilities and the limits of their own rhetorical power. Partial stories also reflect a lack of awareness about the powerful ways that shame—and gendered sexual shame in particular—continues to animate discourse and experiences of many people today, in a social and political climate that remains regressive and unjust for reproducing people, people who identify as women, other minorities, and people doubly marginalized. More fully integrating recorded history with silenced experiences, embodied experiences, and emotional experiences enables an interrogation of the power of an arresting emotion like shame. It is shame, after all, that prompts the affective disorientation expressed by Bazelon—the "weird" feeling of self-blame when being accosted by a "lecherous" person and the sense that even in an effort to recognize violence and injustice "it's not the *least bit* clear" how such recognition will "play out" in public. Shame is more than disorienting. It is toxic when it bolsters silencing, given that the silence of women or of any "traditionally disenfranchised group often goes unremarked upon if noticed at all" (Glenn 2004, 11). In the words of Chanel Miller ("I Am," 2019), the "Emily Doe" who was sexually assaulted by Stanford University student Brock Turner, "Shame, really, can kill you."

As someone writing about gendered experiences, I must pause to clarify my use of terms such as *woman, girl*, and *mother. Woman* denotes any person who uses this label. References throughout this book that imply binary categories of sex are reflections of the recent history from which they are drawn, not my own assumptions about gender fixity. Also in relation to the historical events recounted in this book, the distinction between *girl* and *woman* relates to age but also implicates the politics of representation (e.g., many people who identify as women may feel infantilized if called "girls") and can suggest sexual knowledge and/or experience. Unwed pregnant "girls" may experience simultaneously agency-reducing but otherwise adultlike experiences—especially if they are held solely accountable for their actions. As this book explores, historically these people were often in their teens or early twenties and were punished for being puerile members of a larger patriarchal system. Thus, both *girl* and *woman* seem simultaneously appropriate and unsatisfactory. Given these considerations, *mother* is a particularly apt term.

Enduring Shame revisits women's "recent" reproductive history to understand moments of change, specifically those related to reproductive and sexual autonomy, from the perspective of unwed pregnant people and unwed mothers, a category of women whose independence has long been questioned and whose experiences with reproduction have in the recent past provoked significant intervention and public scrutiny. This recency approach focuses on events that have occurred within one's lifetime "where visibility is inherently imperfect, hindsight and perspective are lacking" (Romano and Potter 2012, 3). Attending to the shifting treatment of unwed mothers (later referred to primarily as pregnant *teens*) through historiography of the recent past offers a unique opportunity to trace the power of emotion—shame, stigma, and blame, specifically—through experiences that have been both private and politicized, whispered about and debated publicly.

The arc of this book illuminates shame's mutability and persistence when directed to women's unsanctioned and defiant, sexual, and fertile bodies. The history I explore in the following pages offers a way of understanding shame's unparalleled and especially rhetorical relationship to women's sexuality and reproduction and the deceptive way that this emotion seems to recede when, as Bazelon suggests, it remains ever present, ever ready to take new forms or be called upon in the name of righteous thought, righteous action. *Righteous* here signifies any belief or position that is thought right or legitimate and connotes a shared set of values around rightness and wrongness that can be thought of as more *doxic,* or reflective of shared public opinion, than religious. With greater understanding of how the communicated and communicable qualities of shame make it not only a felt emotion but an embodied and rhetorical one, people can more fully consider its mis/uses as a weapon of social change. With knowledge of shame as rhetorical, people can also do more than feel disgust when shame is invoked to silence and intimidate. Such awareness can also enable more nuanced and sound responses to comments like those from the former US president, Donald Trump, who, in one instance of being accused of sexual violence, responded "shame on those who make up false stories of assault" (Newburger 2019).

Louise, a woman I interviewed when researching the history of unwed pregnancy and motherhood during an era of extensive secret-keeping and silencing, was similar to other once-unwed mothers; her story revealed that shame was one central (and often the only) factor in upholding the practice of disappearing young, white, unmarried pregnant women and denying their identity as mothers. When I began this project in an effort to learn about a systematically silenced part of women's recent history, I was not expecting to write about shame. But the more I listened to mothers' stories, the more I learned that shame provided a critical rhetorical architecture of practices wherein an unknown number of white, middle-class women secretly bore and then relinquished a child for adoption as part of a socially sanctioned practice meant to erase their status as the mother of a so-called illegitimate child. I also realized that a perceived erosion of shame in the 1970s and later decades was attributed as a primary cause for social change and was considered indicative of how women were responding to cultural shifts that affected their sexual and reproductive lives. This book resists the myth of shame's easy dissipation and uses recent historiography to trace its mutation and endurance.

Other scholars have persuasively made the case for recognizing how unwed and teen mothers were constructed as a problem warranting a collective solution (e.g., Luker 1997; Solinger 2000; Vinson 2018). While I agree with this assessment, additional historiographic lessons can be drawn from a 1970s obsession with diagnosing the "problem" of unwed motherhood and coping with it in ways other than erasure. Despite the alleged dissipation of shame during the 1970s, across this decade the emotion continued to function as a mechanism for responding to and reckoning with social change, especially among women who were particularly vulnerable to its effects. This book focuses most closely on the 1960s and 1970s. I trace a shift from practices of hiding and denying unwed motherhood to more public treatments of teen pregnancy while also attending to the less public, if nevertheless deliberated-upon, practices in various spaces (e.g., schools, courts of law) and among disparate communities during this span of time. In so doing, I catalog ways that shame and blame shift but remain part of affective rhetorical ecologies—lingering in discourses and through logics and practices that not only include articulatable emotional states but also embodied, sensorial, and very real encounters and experiences. These ecologies shaped the material realities of and the perceptions about women who were still considered errant, who still threatened the boundaries of acceptability, and who, for these reasons, elicited the intercession of a nation in flux. These decades of change reveal publics grappling with a "problem" of their own configuration, laboring to reassess and rectify a type of motherhood often thought to be universally unacceptable, and beholden to the rhetorical power of shame that lingered and foreclosed more dialogic, caring, and imaginative responses to this social "issue." Examining closely this one segment of recent reproductive history enables listening to and accounting for a range of experiences and foregrounding the emotional/affective aspects of an increasingly public problem. These tactics are vital to understanding shame's rhetorical power and its persistence. Four fundamental assumptions about rhetoric's relationship to shame ground my analysis:

Rhetorical shame is felt, by which I mean it is effectuated through embodied experiences. Shame has and continues to animate rhetorics (verbal, visual, spatial, etc.) of people living in, or who are perceived to be living in, sexual, reproducing, and (potentially) mothering bodies.

Rhetorical shame engages with a visual continuum whereby invisibility and spectacle are poles that contribute to shame's rhetorical functions: to illuminate, hide, reprimand, foster cohesion, and prompt disidentification.

Rhetorical shame is persuasive (more explicit) and suasive (less explicit, more ambient), and in both cases powerful, which makes responding to it challenging. Doing so requires recognizing and naming its individual and collective instantiations.

Rhetorics of shame primarily operate within a closed rhetorical system. That is, they articulate to an honor-shame order that shifts but does not easily dissolve. What is righteous in one context can be unrighteous in another.

Additionally, shame as an animating variable in recent histories of unwed pregnancy is fueled by an ongoing, if ever-shifting, dialectic of protection and dependency. The "who" or "what" needing protection changes over time and in relation to the threat of women's increasing sexual autonomy and the growing undeniability of sexual realities that illuminate the exclusivity, impracticality, and injustice of righteous reproduction. The rhetorical script for who or what needs protection can be understood in relation to these threats because, in so many instances, what is threatened is dominance and authority of some (the powerful few) over the reproductive lives of others (the many who, individually, are in positions of less power). What is feared is the fully realized ability for all people to have sovereignty over their own sexual and reproductive lives.

The overarching argument of this book is that shame related to sex, gender, and reproducing bodies remains a present, largely misunderstood, and decidedly rhetorical aspect of contemporary life. My historiographic examination of its discursive and felt presence enables theorizing what this emotion *does* rhetorically and how it endures. Sexual shame did not dissolve by the end of the 1960s and has not dissolved today; rather, it is ever shifting, often nefarious, and still present for many women who experience its quieting, sometimes isolating, effects through threats or manifestations of gender-based exploitation or violence. In contemporary dominant Western culture, shame is weaponized in public and political exchange, lingering as a volatile and poorly understood rhetorical affect. Marshalled by rhetors across the bright lines of politics that increasingly divide contemporary discourse, rhetorical uses of shame warrant more critical awareness and deeper understanding of how manifestations of this emotion can mutate but, within wider publics, tend to remain intact and sow division. It is with such awareness that rhetors can cultivate more inclusive, historically informed, dialogic, and affectively attuned positions about reproductive concerns and the intersections of these concerns with other sites of social justice activism.

Telling Stories of Unwed Pregnancy,
Centering Righteous Reproduction

In a 2004 talk to a meeting of the National Abortion Rights Action League (NARAL), author Ursula Le Guin (2016) spoke of life in the years before *Roe v. Wade:* "They asked me to tell what it was like to be twenty and pregnant in 1950 and when you tell your boyfriend you're pregnant, he tells you about a friend of his in the army whose girl told him she was pregnant, so he got all his buddies to come and say, 'We all fucked her, so who knows who the father is?' And he laughs at the good joke" (7). Le Guin goes on to describe what it was like to be "a pregnant girl—we weren't 'women' then—a pregnant college girl who, if her college found out she was pregnant, would expel her, there and then without plea or recourse" (7). These recollections reflect the power of *righteous reproduction*, a term that can describe a social agreement that the army buddies all know. Only certain bodies (white and female) and one relationship status (married) were eligible to produce a sanctioned pregnancy by those upholding norms of white patriarchy. To violate righteous reproduction meant that you could experience severely diminished dignity within a majority white culture; this could be, for instance, being white, pregnant, and unmarried or—in the words of Marlo D. David (2016)—simply "mothering while black" (xi). For a white woman like Le Guin, you could be laughed at, kicked out, hidden. For non-white women, unsanctioned pregnancy could be the basis for losing your right to ever give birth again. Reproduction is often a matter of righteousness because the rightness of some types of pregnancy is often dependent upon a widely held social belief in the wrongness of other types of pregnancy.

Unwed pregnancy and unwed motherhood likely sound to most readers like outmoded ways of referring to what US culture has come to refer to as *teen pregnancy* or *single parenting.* In fact, the language of unwed motherhood fell out of fashion during the 1970s as I discuss in this book. I initially return to the middle of the twentieth century—a time when unmarried and pregnant women, in particular, infrequently had the rhetorical power to counter prevailing practices of dealing with such "illicit" pregnancies. In the years after World War II, the social shame of white unwed pregnancy was connected to elaborate practices of hiding and denying the fact that such pregnancies existed. Such practices are enmeshed with other ways in which heteronormative, patriarchal, white supremacist culture was (re)produced at the time. For example, during this period of national economic prosperity and political dominance, returning veterans wished to reinsert themselves within a workforce that, during the war, had extended to include more African American and white women; upwardly mobile white families who constructed new and exclusive suburban spaces distanced themselves from urban centers, poverty, and racial diversity; and a domestic baby boom aligned with a rise in conspicuous consumption within the "American" home. White culture was manifesting in visual ideals of the white nuclear family that precluded an unmarried and pregnant daughter. The apparatus of "homes for unwed mothers" enabled the visual erasure of unmarried motherhood and provided an avenue to "revirginalization" that was necessary for upholding the purity and sanctity of white motherhood. These mothers themselves, though, were often unable to forget such trauma.

Across the same decades, non-white unwed mothers were typically figured differently. Not only were they ineligible for righteous reproduction, a concept strictly coded in whiteness and within the confines of marriage, but also their reproductive capacities functioned as the foil that could be contrasted on a racialized continuum. Historian Rickie Solinger (2000) explains that Black women were overwhelmingly considered by those subscribing to the supposed superiority of white culture to be both naturally sexual beings and inherent—if always already deviant—mothers. As "permanent victims of their sexuality" (44), Black unwed mothers were less frequently drawn into socially constructed webs of secrecy and hiding, even if they may have experienced keen emotional responses within their communities if they became pregnant while unmarried. Within a majority white culture, however, Black women were often thought to be irredeemably sexualized, thus providing a racialized antithesis to the rhetorical construction of unadulterated white motherhood. While white women were concerned with the shame related to being recognized as pregnant and unmarried, non-white women might have had to contend with other reproductive issues. Coercive or nonconsensual sterilization practices, such as the 1968 forced sterilization of North Carolina resident Elaine Riddick, were publicly debated and put into action as a putative—and tragically permanent—method for managing the "dependency" of poor and "unfit" women (who, in most cases, were non-white, presumed to have a cognitive abnormality, or both). While some non-white women were eligible to go to one of the few mid-century maternity homes that allowed non-white residents, other non-white women kept their children, put their children up for adoption outside of the maternity home/adoption infrastructure, or pursued other options.

With the 1970s came more public ways of engaging the "problem" of unwed pregnancy. Title IX legislation—often recognized as historic for its contribution to women's athletics—was passed by Congress in 1972 and provided the legal basis for pregnant students to stay in school. In the same year, the Supreme Court decision on *Eisenstadt v. Baird* eliminated legal barriers to unmarried persons having access to contraceptives, such as the birth control pill. And just months later, in early 1973, the Supreme Court made abortion effectively legal with the *Roe v. Wade* ruling, providing many women greater reproductive autonomy, if still only through consultation with a doctor. These changes both necessitated more public discussions about women's sexual rights and signaled significant shifts in the prevailing cultural values about sexual purity. On the basis of such developments, the moral regulation of white unwed motherhood —as a violation of righteous reproduction—seemed to be falling away. A closer examination of various discourses of the 1970s, however, illuminates how shame endures through and despite such "advances," and the strenuous rhetorical work needed to actually begin to reorient to its gendered associations and uses.

Such change was also threatening in its potential to undermine once-pervasive codes of sexual purity. The danger latent in this perceived crescendo of liberated, some would say irresponsible, activity was made particularly salient in 1976, with the publication of a comprehensive study of adolescents' sexual activity that identified "teen pregnancy" as a national "epidemic." A nation grappling with an eroding sense of sexual righteousness refocused its attention on the very young woman—now understood largely in relation to the perplexing state of adolescence—especially if she was white. An increasing epidemiological approach would ostensibly forego shame rhetorics for more rational and science-based discourses related to public health, yet shame and blame lingered in the broad public uptake of this renewed examination of teen pregnancy. Across the 1970s, discussions about unrighteous reproduction—the kinds that warranted definition and deliberation in a time of shifting norms— increasingly figured pregnancy outside of marriage as a liability to the state and as an avenue to and/or mark of poverty. Despite earnest efforts to assay and respond to "babies having babies," the public discourse of the late 1970s reflect a sexual double-standard, often steeped in notions that reflect the values of white, normative culture, that continued to cast young women as responsible for their unruly reproductive bodies and their consequences.

This book traces women's experiences, perceptions, and feelings through this recent history of unwed pregnancy to explain righteous reproduction as a gendered, racialized, class- and ability-inflected purity code that took shape by mid-century and that has continued implications for how people understand, talk about, and advocate for issues of reproduction, pregnancy, and motherhood. I move in a mostly chronological manner through two decades to slowly account for a period of great transformation in which ostensibly private practices that functioned as open secrets gave way to public reckonings with sexual desire, reproductive rights, and related questions of agency, vulnerability, and responsibility. While in some ways this is an examination of legal, medical, and moral change related to young women and reproductive politics, the rhetorical construction of age and age's relationship to desire, reproductive possibility, innocence, disability, and rhetorical empowerment threads through this historiography. The role of biological age and relative maturity (ideas that are largely shaped by racialized notions of normalcy and deviance) advance and recede through chapters that examine political shifts that sometimes apply to most (perhaps even all) women and those that are more focused on key subsets of women (such as school-age girls). Despite these somewhat interwoven aspects of the book, I consistently identify righteous reproduction as a central normativizing force—a claim that suggests several distinct findings and possibilities.

First, righteous reproduction as a coherent cultural logic helps explain differential ways of figuring, responding to, and acting upon various reproductive and pregnant bodies in earlier decades. In simpler terms, it explains the beliefs that undergird what seems to be logical and right. I rely here on Krista Ratcliffe's (2006) notion of *cultural logic*, which names the culturally specific, often tacit, sense of the right and the logical among a group of people at a particular moment in time (10). A cultural logic explains why some pregnancies (e.g., those of unwed white women) were likely to be intervened upon—hidden, denied, and (imperfectly) erased. It also explains why other reproducing bodies were not subjected to such elision but could still be managed. White married women having babies were models of motherhood and sanctioned reproduction so long as this motherhood performed submissiveness and domesticity. Non-white women having babies outside of marriage were less eligible for the "protections" of hiding and erasure but were often considered deserving of other public intervention and management because of a perceived need for authorities to regulate their unwieldy reproductive potential. Today, it can be perplexing to grapple with the extensiveness of practices of hiding and child surrender that was a familiar and normalized feature of life in the United States (and other parts of the world).[2] Recognizing reproductive righteousness as a coherent code of gendered, racialized, and class-oriented sexual purity aids in revisiting stories and experiences of these earlier times and coming to terms with how they operated logically in the recent past. In revisiting this history, I more fully examine how rhetorics of shame animate much of this discourse and articulate the complex rhetorical network of language, affect, and embodiment through which shame moves and that moves people toward various actions and beliefs.

Second, righteous reproduction expands a rhetorical understanding of the discursive power of two identities, *woman* and *mother,* as negotiated, politically potent, and normalizing (or normalized). This study of young women as unrighteous mothers deepens an understanding of the rhetorical force of these terms. More specifically, righteous reproduction contributes to Lindal Buchanan's (2013) theory of a "code of motherhood" whereby *Mother* and *Woman* are terms, concepts, and identities that function on a continuum in public discourse and public life. Buchanan's theory demonstrates how *Mother* functions as a god term—a term generally embraced and elevated as being especially positive—in everyday discourses that signifies "a myriad of positive associations, including children, love, protection, home, nourishment, altruism, morality, religion, self-sacrifice, strength, the reproductive body, the private sphere, and the nation" (8). *Woman*, operating as the opposite devil term—one that shares a nefarious cultural connotation—conjures negative associations: "childlessness, self-centeredness, work, materialism, hysteria, irrationality, the sensual/sexual body, and the public sphere" (8). Righteous reproduction reflects the axes of this larger continuum, and in the case of unwed and teenage pregnancy becomes the basis for arguing over the effects and dangers of women's increasing sexual autonomy and less regulated reproducing bodies. The increasing attention on a crisis of *youth* illustrates that public schools were a primary site of reckoning but also that improperly monitored *girls becoming women* were a primary threat to the sanctity of "Mother." An age-inflected social crisis of "babies having babies" warranted righteous oversight of some young women (those who could be rehabilitated and contribute to a capitalist society), while these increasingly "rational" and ostensibly dispassionate mediations trafficked in some of the negative connotations Buchanan links to *Woman*.

Indeed, the age of young mothers and potential young mothers—young people understood in relation to a constructed state of pre-pregnancy—justified intervention by the body politic, whether that be in the name of reconfiguring righteous reproducing bodies or terminating the reproductive capability of those reproducing bodies (poor, non-white) who were deemed unlikely to reproduce in ways the majority culture sanctioned. Such intervention happened at the nexus of several factors that coalesced around young women. These factors include increased access to sex (actual, imagined, and feared, through access to oral contraceptives or abortion, for instance), less socially deterministic codes of desire (which were expressed as the diminished stigma and shame of premarital sex and its consequences for women), and uneven and emergent approaches to cultivating epistemologies about sex (e.g., through fledgling public school sex education programs). In short, as possibilities for women's sexual autonomy manifested, varied forms of age-oriented righteousness became the panacea for unfettered sexual sovereignty. Rather than encouraging women to embrace and navigate their shifting relationship with sex with the goal of increased self-efficacy, righteousness *reappears* to tamp down anxieties and guard the preferences of those who feared and/or opposed women's sexual autonomy.

Finally, righteous reproduction as a gendered, raced, and classed concept aids in conceptualizing reproductive dignity and its historical curtailments—a concept that continues to be overseen and deliberated on. Dignity is too frequently the province of politicized publics rather than being an inherent quality and right, imminent in all people. Reproductive righteousness can function as a critical intersectional tool for identifying and connecting instances of indignity —often sites of rhetorical shaming and blaming as well as material violences— that might otherwise be hard to locate and link through extant frames for understanding women's recent history and ongoing struggles. For instance, such a frame enables exploring the privileges and violences experienced by white unwed mothers of the 1950s and 1960s as distinct from but not unconnected to the ongoing child removal policies of the US foster care system that affect Black children in ways that Dorothy Roberts has likened to apartheid (Threadcraft 2018, 170). Righteousness as a frame applied across time can shine light on legacies of injustice and their manifestations today. It can, for example, support critical awareness-building through rhetorical analysis of such vexing issues as the crises of sexual assault in higher education and the ways that this site of violence continues to be addressed through victim-blaming. It can aid in articulating something as pervasive but amorphous as rape culture and grappling with the lasting effects of sexual assault. While not the only tool necessary to address ongoing issues related to sexual politics and violences, righteous reproduction as a rhetorical resource can assist in critically navigating such sites of discord past and present.

Why Rhetoric and Shame?

I use the term *rhetorics of shame* to describe a confluence of rhetorical, or persuasive and epistemological, forces: discursive, affective, spatial, visual, material. These rhetorics cohere around shame as an experience described by contemporary philosophers: shame is a reactive experience of a person "unable to honor the demands consubstantial with . . . certain [social] values" (Deonna, Rodogno, and Teroni 2012, xii). Shame is an evaluation of the self that determines that self somehow unworthy or degraded (7). In more everyday terms, shame is the overwhelming and deeply personal feeling that one experiences, in the mind, in the body, and on the surface of the body, that acutely registers a perceived failure or disappointment in the eyes of another, even if that other is not present or not even an actual person. Shame is an often-private feeling that can shape our thoughts and actions whether they be private or public.

My conception of rhetorical shame does not rely on the fixity of moral codes but rather on the flux of any "system of sociality" (Mendible 2016, 1) and the system's rhetorical qualities. Although shame has been explained by psychologists with special attention to personal feeling and cognition, scholars press to understand shame as an intersubjective and embodied experience and thus to move beyond individual, primarily cognitive, explanations of the emotion. Political philosopher Jill Locke (2016) captures this need for more social theorizing: "even as shame involves a set of generally agreed-upon psychological and bodily sensations, it has no clear ontology" (19). Shame functions within a thoroughly social milieu; what is shameful (or not) depends upon agreed-upon and potentially ever-changing standards. Additionally, the work of shame—the blush that burns one's skin, the desire to hide from others when feeling ashamed (downcast eyes, hiding one's face in one's hands, an actual hiding away from others)—results from the idea of being seen and the desire to not be seen. In these ways, shame functions as a rhetorical emotion; yet to date there has not been a sustained exploration of rhetorics of shame. Melissa V. Harris-Perry (2011), who has theorized the emotion in relation to social history, argues compellingly for locating shame as a central part of Black Americans' political and social experience and an acute experience for African American women, in particular. Whereas her project identifies "mechanism[s] for the production of shame" (111) and the effects of racialized shame culture, questions remain as to how shame works rhetorically, as a socially and personally powerful emotion that is both communicated and communicable.

In the chapters that follow, I explain how shame is a persuasive and social emotion, how it plays a role in public decision-making (or avoidance), and how its rhetorical power can remain unrecognized or mischaracterized if we do not sufficiently understand the emotion's operations in public. The history I share demonstrates shame's power to overshadow knowledge-seeking, deliberation, and perspective-building—its ability to overpower other rhetorical forms and ways of being. This examination of the increasingly public and allegedly rationalized discourses and practices related to unwed pregnancy illustrates that an honor-shame order can shift but does not easily dissolve. In my conclusion, I argue that an honor-shame order is a closed rhetorical system that impedes the normalizing of the sexual sovereignty of all women.

Although these considerations hew closely to the "traditional" understandings of rhetoric as persuasion in civic and/or public contexts, I engage with the topic of shame through a feminist lens. My understanding of rhetoric is fundamentally shaped by theories of rhetoric's relationship to gender and power as well as its being experienced through embodiment and relevant to communication about material, human bodies. I look to Cheryl Glenn's (1997) foundational work in regendering rhetoric as a reminder that rhetoric "always inscribes the relation of language and power at a particular moment" (1–2). Although this book recounts histories of women, my feminist rhetorical approach compels me to ask how shame functions in sites of uneven power—unevenness that stems from gendered expectations, economic disparities, racism, and the like. Rhetoric is a tool for indexing and understanding how these sites of social inequality come to exist, how they retain persuasive power, and how they change (or not). Additionally, I advocate approaching these relationships through the concept of rhetorics of shame because doing so enables me to take seriously the relationship between rhetoric and bodies, since shame is an embodied emotion and because rhetorics of shame are often deployed in relation to bodies that fail to conform to some expectation of bodily honor (e.g., they are incorrectly pregnant, they are dis/abled, they are "problematically" asexual, they are atypically sexual). Jay Timothy Dolmage (2014), who argues for recognizing rhetoric as the "strategic study of the circulation of power through communication," has cultivated this understanding through an explicit focus on the body's centrality to rhetoric (3). *Enduring Shame* dives into a history of unsanctioned pregnancy and reproductive (in)justice in order to observe the "tensions, trials, and trouble" (Dolmage 2014, 16) experienced by those people who, because their bodies were understood as deviant in light of righteous reproduction, were shamed.

Shame has been of recent and developing interest among feminist scholars and contributes to what Clara Fischer (2018) refers to as a "'new school' of feminism made up of affect theorists and new materialists" (372). This larger turn toward affect and materiality invokes concerns of "the body, affect, and emotion, and generally present[s] feeling-states as embodied phenomena" (372). As such, throughout this book I reference shame as emotion and as affect, and I construct contexts that I refer to as *affective rhetorical ecologies*. As feminist rhetoricians also turn to affect, materiality, and the related questions of posthumanism, new questions about agency, and agency's relationship to gender and power, arise. This book values affect as a nondiscursive, embodied, and everyday emotional engagement that plays a significant role in rhetorical processes of gendering and the rhetorical artifacts that emerge when these processes are called into question.

Several aspects of shame—a notoriously complex and vexing emotion to study—provide a basis from which I build my analysis. Although early psychological work has focused largely on the distinction between guilt (a result of bad action) and shame (a result of personal failing; Scheff 2000), ongoing and cross-disciplinary theory provides additional insight on this emotion that is helpful in thinking about its mutability in public discourse and rhetorical practice. The culturally attuned work of scholars—especially queer theorists—has helped to expand the study of shame beyond the discipline of psychology and, particularly, individual psychology. Increasingly, scholars from various disciplines see shame as contributing to group identity formation—noting how it accretes to form a "collective politics of shame" (Ahmed 2004, 102) and how the emotion performs "cultural labor" that, in part, "attempts to mark and contain fluid boundaries" such as those of national and group identities (Mendible 2016, 9). As I trace shame's presence in the shifting practices related to and rhetorical framings of unwed pregnancy, I explore shame's perceptibility through physical bodies, the paradox of shame being felt individually but operating as a social emotion, and the unique relationship of shame to gendered processes and experiences.

Feminist scholars have argued that women are more prone to experiencing shame than men (Bartky 1990; Manion 2003; Johnson and Moran 2013) and that because of the persuasive logics that contribute to gendered shame culture, women can be understood as being "schooled by the strictures of shame" (Stenberg 2018, 122). The rise of Christianity in Europe involved trying to diminish the presumed power women had because of "erotic attraction," a goal pursued by "making sexuality an object of shame" (Federici 2014, 37). Shame as a learned part of gendered publicity has most recently been considered by Locke, who examines the historical legacy of *pudeur,* or feminine modesty. Locke (2016) refers to *pudeur* as a "virtuous restraint," (116) and contends that by the nineteenth century, the concept was "very much a call to action" for women who were not only expected to show restraint and demureness themselves, but also to teach this modesty to others, thus bolstering the attitude through its defense and reproduction (117). The long shadow of shame's relationship to gendered expectations for public presence (or invisibility) and the rhetorical implications of this tradition serve as an exigence for this study.

Mapping Shame's Rhetorical Terrain

Because shame is a social emotion and because its movement is infrequently linear, it is useful to account for how this emotion functions rhetorically in the specific historiography of this book. This shame landscape is informed by a controlling cultural logic, operates within an affective rhetorical ecology, is shaped by a primary dialectical tension of rightness and wrongness, and features a resulting shame- or blame-based rhetorical response. I use the term *terrain* purposefully, to gesture toward shame's often spatial, visual, embodied, and always experiential characteristics. Although a topographical concept, I invoke a sense of *being within* a context both material and dimensional.

Subsequent chapters investigate salient moments in the recent history of unwed pregnancy to explain how shame operates rhetorically and among stakeholders participating in—or implicated by—the conversations at hand. This overview of shame's rhetorical terrain provides groundwork for articulating a four-part theory of rhetorical shame.

1. *Radial rhetorics of shame* names how shame functioned privately within families as a conduit for erasing unrighteous (young, white, and unwed) mothers through much of the 1960s.
2. *Stigmatizing rhetorics of contagious bodily shame* articulates the contagious threat experienced in, on, and through gendered bodies that warranted containment, particularly notable in school spaces.

3. *Sticky rhetorics of persistent shame* draws on Sara Ahmed's (2004) notion of emotional "stickiness" to name the process by which shame-based anxieties seep into discourses (here, juridical and technical) where sexual autonomy and freedoms *seem* to be codified through legal and scientific "progress" but are paradoxically undercut based on gendered shame identities. These rhetorics function counterintuitively to inhibit agency cultivation and instead "grant" agency in a contingent form that can later be eroded or rescinded; alternative rhetorics do more durable work of affectively realigning away from gendered shame.

4. *Shifting rhetorics of public blame* disguises shame-orientations through narratives of public wellbeing (here, public health) that corral shame and fix it onto the body in public, rendering it eligible for ostensibly nonmoralizing, deliberative intervention.

My historiographic examination of discursive patterns and practices debunks a lingering myth that women's sexual shame dissipated in/through the 1970s, maps shame's rhetorical operation over time, and illuminates its tenacity through a period of significant change.

Listening to History: A Feminist Rhetorical Historiographic Approach

Why turn to a recent history of unwed and teen pregnancy? Why examine this recent past (i.e., experienced by those who are still living) through the lens of feminist historiography, a methodology for writing rhetoric's ever-more-capacious histories and for exploring the rhetorical quality of any historical account? Historiographic methodology prompts rhetoricians to ask themselves "what constitutes the history of rhetoric, how to study it, and rhetoric's role in forming and promoting the common good" (Agnew, Gries, and Stuckey 2011, 110). Rhetorical historiography has been taken up by various scholars including feminist rhetoricians who are eager to expand the perspectives and voices accounted for within rhetorical studies and to use rhetorical theory and analysis to explore sites of power inequities and "processes of gendering" (Enoch 2013). Resisting the notion that rhetorical historiography can ever be complete, given that it is, by definition, partial, Glenn (2018) insists that "feminist scholars must continue to intervene in rhetorical histories, especially when their interpolations invigorate our understandings of rhetoric's capacities and infinite instantiations across time and space" (105). This project takes up shared feminist historiographic goals articulated by Jessica Enoch: recovering women's voices, identifying recurring patterns within women's rhetorical history (here patterns of shaming), contextualizing women's rhetorical contributions (or exclusions, as this recent history suggests), analyzing traditional rhetoric's oversight of some "female or feminized rhetors," and creating rhetorical theories that "more equitably reinscribe women's rhetorical participation" (quoted in Royster and Kirsch 2012, 103). But in addition to these interconnected goals, a historiography of unwed pregnancy uses this methodology to account for women's *rhetorical power* in relation to their sexual and reproductive identities.

As a project that focuses on *rhetorical* history, this book lives somewhere in the space between "recovery"—here a term for the feminist rhetorical aim of identifying and learning from women who have been excluded from the scholarly rhetorical tradition—and the goal of creating "a fuller picture" of women's lives as does Saidiya Hartman (Okeowo 2020). That is, I rely on evidence and archive where I am able (even as I reject the power-laden, salvationlike implications of the word *recovery*), and in several key places I lean toward the speculative (doing so with transparency and caution). More centrally, this book engages with the "fundamental rhetorical issues" articulated by Glenn (2004): "who speaks, who remains silent, who listens, and what those listeners can do" (23). Listening to once-unwed mothers' stories of being silenced and told to forget about their identity as mothers supports the long-held goal of feminist rhetoricians to expand the horizon of whose rhetorical experiences scholars pay attention to, record, and try to understand in relation to issues of gender and power. I am informed by Rickie Solinger's definition of *reproductive politics* as a term originally used by second-wave feminists that can be used as a heuristic to ask "*Who has power over matters of pregnancy and its consequences?*" (3; emphasis in original). Solinger (2007) identifies six ideas that animate the "arena" (4) of reproductive politics: its relationship to "solving social problems" (4), its relevance in "responding to women's everyday practices" (9), its centrality to "contesting the meaning of womanhood" (12), its preoccupation with "making 'private' choices in public contexts" (14), the need for a historical approach to the subject that "track[s] change over time" (17), and the assertion that there can never be a "single history" of reproduction because of the social and political influences in understanding and managing this biological event (21).

A historiography of *pregnancy* centers pregnancy's physicality, its ubiquity, and its significance to gendering norms. This book takes seriously Elizabeth Flietz's (2015) argument that focusing on the body is "central" to investigations of women's rhetorics even when rhetorical scholars must identify new historiographic methods and approaches to do such work (34–36). I hope that revisiting stories of some women's experiences in relation to pregnancy and shame, while adding to feminist examinations of everyday and politicized experiences, can complement other rhetorical investigations of "bodies in rhetorical practice" (Chávez 2018, 245).

Additionally, the stories and discourses I examine in this book, particularly their affective valences, help to reveal "rhetoric[s] of normalization" (Enoch

2005, 16) about gender and reproduction and ways "normalcy is used to control bodies" (Dolmage and Lewiecki-Wilson 2010, 24). Too often publics configure progress narratives of reproductive attainment that deny the experience of many people—narratives that are so gains-focused that they promote a false sense of the stability and self-evidence of all, or even most, people's reproductive autonomy. These normalizing rhetorics should figure more prominently in academic and public accounts of women's recent histories of sexual and reproductive agency. It is an overreliance on partial and progress-oriented retellings that contributes to feelings of not only anger but also frustration, confusion, and despair among those who fear a reversal or rollback of reproductive gains by contemporary political and judicial leadership. Such retellings also reify the notion that past "gains"—if not reversed—sufficiently account for the range of exigences people experience in relationship to reproduction. Rhetorical shame has been effectuated to silence or otherwise rhetorically constrain many people, including those who identify as women. Attention to the way rhetorical mechanisms of injustice take hold and seem reasonable is the sort of rhetorical work Enoch contends is necessary for feminist historiographers examining discourses of the twentieth century (17, 24). Additionally, I heed Jay Dolmage and Cynthia Lewiecki-Wilson's call for bringing disability studies' attention to constructions of bodily normalcy, deviancy, and "enfreakment" to feminist rhetorical projects because this approach "provides an essential critical perspective on the ways knowledge is created, categories are enforced, and bodies are valued across time periods and geographies" (38).

Identifying logics of normalization is of critical concern to understanding this history for several reasons. First, logics of normalcy resulted in once-unwed women being hidden and their experiences systematically silenced—a practice that does not have a regular place in public rememberings of recent reproductive history. Second, logics of *racial* normalcy (as an expression of white supremacy) and *age-based* normalcy have significantly contributed to practices and discussions about which pregnancies are considered acceptable and which are marked as illicit at any given moment in time. And finally, logics of normalcy related to recent histories of reproductive politics continually center the experience of white women and figure reproductive change through the lens of judicial, technological, and policy outcomes that are widely understood to be about "choice" and reproductive autonomy. The power that these codifications exert over shared stories and understandings of reproductive politics has resulted in a relatively thin and partial narrative that has for too long been accepted despite feminists' activist and scholarly efforts. A public reliance on this framing of reproductive agency granted (and potentially taken away) through judicial and policy mechanisms has discouraged interweaving marginalized histories (e.g., of unwed white women, of Black and brown women, of sterilization abuses) into more widely circulating, fully representative narratives of the reproductive "gains" of the 1970s and later. I agree with Solinger (2007) that accounting for various histories "is crucial to the project of showing that sex and pregnancy is more than a biological event" and that women "have lived reproductive lives under variously constrained or capacious circumstances" depending on social and historical factors (21, 25). This book expands this "project" by demonstrating how reproductive normalcy is rhetorically constructed and by exploring how shame contributes to the maintenance of normalcy as legible and reproduced (discursively, affectively, and physically).

Doing this historiographic work and tracing the ways that various women's sense of rhetorical and sexual agency shifted (but did not become fully realized) after shame ostensibly gave way to less moralistic and public discussions of reproduction also aligns with Sarah Hallenbeck's (2015) efforts to trace "gender differences" that "are transformed through shifts in the material networks that women inhabit" (xvi). In this study, I consider material networks to be the wide-ranging rhetorical ecologies—affective, visual, spatial, and embodied—that are central to the varied stories of women's reproduction during these decades of change. In this way I take up Hallenbeck's claim that "gender socialization emerges from historically situated contexts of activity" (xxi) and respond to her call to appreciate how "rhetorical effort both emerge[s] and reverberate[s]" within activity networks (xviii). As a study of a changing landscape over time, this book extends feminist historiographic attempts to shift away from individual sites of rhetorical production and a humanistic assumption of coherent subjectivity and agency.

In sum, this book asks: *How might rhetorics of shame be understood as a gendered phenomenon through the study of one portion of women's recent history?* By exploring this question, I not only contribute to ongoing efforts at feminist rhetorical recovery, but also posit a rhetorical theory of shame that can be used across other sites of historiography, analysis, and rhetorical criticism. It is my hope that such feminist rhetorical work contributes to the larger, necessarily coalitional, project of rhetorical feminism by asking "what possibilities might we imagine and work to create for a more equitable future for us all" and by laboring toward answers that examine "our present-past" not merely to "confront what has become outlived (the waste and foolishness) but to discover the potential of what is living within ourselves" (Glenn 2018, 196).

Learning from History: Reproductive Justice and Rhetorical Feminism

Enduring Shame focuses on the social shift from unjust practices such as hiding some pregnant and unwed bodies and sterilizing some people to more public, juridical, legal, and medically oriented ways of ostensibly providing women with greater reproductive autonomy. Though this historical shift *does* relate to activist efforts to gain bodily entitlements, I am purposefully choosing to *not* situate this history as one of "reproductive rights" because of the limitations such terminology perpetuates. Instead, this book works to align with the focus, goals, and intersectional methodology of reproductive justice, a more comprehensive, inclusive, and just way of addressing issues related to reproductive politics.

Tracing and theorizing rhetorics of shame allows me to present reproductive righteousness as relevant to intersectional feminist inquiry that can yoke seemingly different experiences of reproduction in ways that I hope do not minimize any one story but rather offer perspective through telling many stories. To enact rhetorical feminism with this caveat in mind, I am casting this history as one that relates not only to unwed or teenage mothers *as mothers* or *as pregnant women* but as a historiography that can—and should—be situated within a larger context of reproductive politics. More specifically, in writing this book, I have made an effort to learn from and heuristically apply ideas from the robust activist theory of reproductive justice. As a methodology, a movement, and an "emergent radical theory," reproductive justice represents the intellectual *and* activist, always-coalitional work of Black women and other communities of color (Ross et al. 2017, 13). As an approach for "thinking about the experience of reproduction," reproductive justice "splices *reproductive rights* with *social justice"* in order to engage in meaning-making and activism that extends beyond the pro-choice versus pro-life debate that dominates contemporary public discourse about reproduction (Ross and Solinger 2017, 9; emphasis in original).

The rich history of the reproductive justice movement is detailed in both *Undivided Rights: Women of Color Organize for Reproductive Justice* (Silliman et al. 2004) and *Radical Reproductive Justice: Foundations, Theory, Practice, Critique* (Ross et al. 2017). These texts carefully account for the vast number of and varied types of people who have worked, before and since 1994, to create a needed "paradigm shift" for ending reproductive oppression (Leonard 2017, 39). An initial group of twelve Black organizers working in reproductive health and reproductive rights movements met that year with the aim of finding ways to center the voices and the needs of Black women in the realm of reproductive politics (46). Drawing from earlier activists and other people of color enabled expansion of this early collaboration, and reproductive justice as a concept began to come into being in ways that exceeded what the original founders had imagined (45). Some of those contributing to this broadening were members of the Latina Roundtable on Health and Reproductive Rights, the Black Women's Health Imperative, the National Latina Health Organization, the Native American Women's Health Education Resource Center, Asian Pacific Islanders for Choice, and Project Azuka member and AIDS activist Juanita Williams (Strickler and Simpson 2017, 50; Zavella 2020, 2). In 1997, several years after a reproductive justice framework had been articulated, the organization that would become SisterSong Women of Color Reproductive Justice Collective was formed to galvanize people and proactively organize for reproductive needs in ways that were not being met by mainstream, white feminist reproductive rights efforts (Strickler and Simpson 2017, 51). By 2003, SisterSong held its first national conference, "inviting other women of color and white allies to build a concerted movement" (Leonard 2017, 47).

Reproductive justice has crystalized around three key human rights: "(1) the right *not* to have a child; (2) the right to *have* a child; and (3) the right to *parent* children in safe and healthy environments" (Ross and Solinger 2017, 9; emphasis in original). Additionally, reproductive justice "demands sexual autonomy and gender freedom for every human being" (65). As Loretta J. Ross and Rickie Solinger argue, these goals are "not difficult to define or remember"; achieving them is the challenge (65). Variously throughout this book, I consider one or more of these three fundamental rights in my historiographic inquiry, using them heuristically to frame my approach to engaging with the given moment of the recent past that I am investigating.

Critically, to understand reproductive justice as "neither an oppositional nor a peacemaking framework" but rather as "an emergent radical theory that reframes" problems (Ross and Solinger 2017, 113), one must also understand the centrality of human rights in the movement's theory of change. The international human rights framework supports holistic and inclusive work toward justice as it models a "sturdy, moral, political, and legal structure through which reproductive justice goals may eventually be accomplished" (79). This comprehensive approach moves beyond the limited, change-by-degree, zero-sum, and often geopolitically tethered tack of other legal and rights-based frameworks, such as those enabled by the US Constitution. In this book, I work to adopt this approach to consider the affordances of a basic, that is fundamental and fully inclusive, rights orientation—one that also envisions a "dialectical, or interactive, relationship between individual and group rights" (84). My use of the term *sovereignty* alongside the more typically individuating word *autonomy* in the book is meant to convey the goal of reproductive freedoms that are not *separate* from networks of care but, rather, enacted through them. Additionally, the foundational values of this human rights orientation, that "all fertile persons and persons who reproduce and become parents require a *safe* and *dignified* context for these most fundamental human experiences" (Ross and Solinger 2017, 9; emphasis added) are woven throughout this project. Comprehensive human rights, including the right to experience (or choose not to experience) sex and reproduction with safety and dignity, are rich and illuminating notions for exploring and explaining notions of righteousness in recent decades and in the case of unwed or teen pregnancy. The reproductive justice movement's intentional and positive engagement with young people to whom such rights also extend and whose voices and perspectives are considered valuable (Zavella 2020) is another prominent influence on my investigation.

Also important to understand (especially in relation to the scope of this book) is that reproductive justice is not only a concern of women *as reproducing beings* but is, rather, a concern for overlapping sites of oppression that delimit women's ability to enjoy freedoms related to sex, reproduction, non/motherhood, and parenting. The movement wishes to explore and act upon the linkages that exist between reproduction and other issues of social justice such as poverty, immigration, criminalization, environmental degradation, and violence (Price 2010, 43). In her work to demonstrate how all politics are related to reproductive politics by leveraging the questions and approaches of reproductive justice, historian Laura Briggs makes a bold case for the need to attend to the labor implications of reproduction in the United States. "The time to do reproductive labor is being shut down as a result of broad political and economic changes that have transformed the relationship of business, government, and households," writes Briggs (2017, 7–8). These economic considerations figure into my investigation, especially as I consider the shame-laden US public discourses related to state dependency that circulated in the 1970s.

Similarly expansive in scope is a June 2018 SisterSong Instagram post featuring artwork by the Repeal Hyde Art Project (fig. 1). SisterSong proclaimed that "keeping families together is reproductive justice," a message in response to the Trump administration's decision to separate children and parents when immigrant families arrived at the US border seeking asylum. The caption further explains that "Taking children away from their parents and tearing families apart is state sanctioned violence. #familiesbelongtogether." As a unified text, the image, words, and hashtag illustrate that reproductive justice extends beyond the temporal or social constraints often associated with reproductive issues and instead identifies how gendered sites of oppression directed to mothers, nonmothers, and/or families are part of this movement—oppressions that are relevant to the recent history explored in this book.

Significant to my engagement with the reproductive justice framework alongside feminist rhetorical historiography, it is important to note that reproductive justice as a site of knowledge-making and activism distinguishes itself from some longstanding feminist interests and attunements. This coalitional effort is explicitly intent on "undermin[ing] the hegemonic narrative of the women's movement that continues to exclude [the] voices and neglect [the] needs" of people of color (Roberts, Ross, and Kuumba 2005, 94). The movement should be understood as different from the narrower second-wave feminist

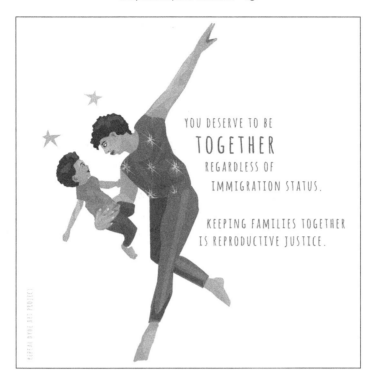

Figure 1. Megan J. Smith, illustration of reproductive justice for the Repeal Hyde Art Project, 2019. Courtesy of Megan J. Smith.

(read: white, heteronormative, and privileged) focus on protecting women's legal access to abortion. This distinction stems from, in part, reproductive justice's explicit commitment to critiquing epistemologies that shore up white supremacy and capitalism—a perspective explored most fully in chapter 3 of this book, where I interrogate macronarratives of reproductive change. Because reproductive justice theory draws upon and extends critical race theory and critical feminist theory, its "cornerstone," according to Ross (2017), is an analysis of white supremacy (173). White allies are invited to engage reproductive justice theory "with integrity" by "question[ing] neoliberal discourses about individual rights and the marketplace of choices denied to the vulnerable members of our society" (223). Doing so carries forth reproductive justice's methodological pursuit of fully conceptualizing reproduction as a site of privilege and the implications of whiteness at this site. My focus on unwed pregnancy upholds reproductive justice's commitment to "plac[e] vulnerable people in the center of [its] lens" as a methodological step in "help[ing] people understand the relationship between white supremacy and white privilege"

(176). This approach foregrounds interdependent and intersectional analysis, exploring the "complex relationship between lived experiences and knowledge production by challenging false binaries and false solutions" through cross-disciplinary synthesis (172).

Finally, a preferred movement strategy for reproductive justice theory building, advocacy, and activism is storytelling, a method used to raise awareness and communicate the meaning that communities make for themselves. Storytelling has helped reproductive justice activists and scholars record the experiences of women of color and other marginalized people facing oppression and share these stories as a form of consciousness-raising (Price 2010, 50). As methodological commitment, the rhetorical form of storytelling-as-activism supports the movement's larger goals of working on behalf of all people, operating outside of a discursive framework of reproductive choice, and validating the experiences of a range of people facing different varieties of reproductive oppression. Additionally, *interlinking* stories and perspectives is especially useful in rendering white privilege visible, given that "downstream consequences of upstream racism" are not always self-evident or apparent (Ross et al. 2017, 25).

I thus rely on story and methods of interlinking throughout this book, pairing reproductive justice approaches with rhetorical methodological work of Indigenous scholars such as Ellen Cushman (2016), Rachel Jackson (2017), and Malea Powell (2012) as well as critical race and cultural rhetorics scholars (Cedillo et al. 2018; Martinez 2020). Jackson draws upon the work of both Cushman and Powell as well as upon her own ethnographic research to make the case for using story as a "decolonial method for disrupting hegemonic abstraction and dislocated frames by building and strengthening community identity" (2017, 499). Collectively, these scholars practice Indigenous ways of thinking, knowing, and doing in order to advocate for the value of understanding story as a site of collaboration that is emplaced, localized, community oriented, and transhistorical. The rhetorical value of story taken up by these scholars aligns with the commitment to story of reproductive justice activists who seek to listen to those who face reproductive oppressions and who explore freedoms, possibilities, and varied ways of knowing. Doing so fosters hope and understanding as well as action in response to interlocking forms of injustice.

Coda: On Limitations and Possibilities

My work to learn from and engage with reproductive justice theory stems from my sense that people like me (white people who experience multiple forms of privilege) can make some ethical and useful justice-oriented contribution to reproductive politics. This notion aligns with my understanding that despite the history of the movement, reproductive justice "does not only apply to women of color" but is a flexible space for learning from others and working in coalition—always with mindfulness and toward shared goals (Ross et al. 2017, 23). Relatedly, a major concern of mine in writing this book—and in working on this project over a span of years and a changing cultural and political landscape—is how my arguments address shame in relation to race. Throughout the book, I have made claims about reproductive righteousness acting as a morality-identity-activity matrix whereby normalcy is upheld. Such "normalcy" articulates to many factors of reproductive righteousness: gendered notions of sexual purity (an ideal) and sexual shame (purity's antithesis); the presumed superiority of whiteness; homogeneity of a sanctioned family structure (i.e., the two-parent nuclear family); the anti-dependency bias of neoliberalism; and the primacy of (hetero)sexuality. Examining shame as a rhetorical and embodied phenomenon related to reproductive righteousness presents an opportunity to learn about the public uses of this emotion in relation to private and public decisions that have had lasting effects on individuals, families, and communities—and to do so with the hope of accounting more fully for how emotion is operationalized in support of agendas that perpetuate hierarchy, division, and injustice. I have worked to consider the experiences of a variety of women who were pregnant and unmarried in this recent history, and I rely on perspectives of interviewees—primarily in chapter 1, given its focus on a secreted history. Readers will notice, however, that there are far more first-person accounts of such experiences from white women than from non-white women. This disparity has been the most complex aspect of my research and writing; indeed, it is one that I have grappled with through various iterations of the project. Although I address race (and many of these other factors of normalcy) in each chapter, it is important for me to provide in this introduction a more encompassing account for my decisions and ways of thinking about race, in particular.

Most generally, I am aware that the invitational research design of my work depends on people choosing to share intimate personal stories that often, but do not necessarily, relate to shame feelings. Such disclosure is entirely voluntary, but it necessitates interviewees trusting me as well as desiring that someone like me (a middle-class, not-yet middle-age, white researcher) hear and learn from their personal story. As a recent anthology collaboratively edited by Tarana Burke and Brené Brown (2021) highlights, interpersonal discussions of shame that relate to race (or that are explored from the perspective of someone not in a majority position) can be especially fraught. Burke, a long-time friend of Brown's prior to their collaborative writing about shame, admits the worry she felt in broaching these topics. As Burke explains, "my lived experience told me that the entire idea and experience of vulnerability feels like a very dangerous place to play, an unsafe thing to even consider or think about as a Black person in this country" (xvii). Another contributor to the collection,

Tanya Denise Fields, shares her perspective on the challenge of being a Black person who openly discusses feelings of vulnerability: "I believed that in doing so I would seem weak, stupid, and fraudulent," and that disclosure "would seem like an admission to the very loud detractors that I was in fact a walking mess of a stereotype" (2021, 27). While these writers do not speak for all people of color, reading their perspectives encourages recognizing the extraordinarily delicate contexts in which stories of negative emotions like shame might be shared, in which lived experiences and ways of knowing might be offered, all in the hope of cultivating understanding within, and possibly across, communities.

It may not be surprising, then, that finding opportunity to engage with nonwhite people who have had an experience with unwed pregnancy has been challenging. I recruited for participants across several regions of the United States including the upper Midwest, the Northeast, and the upper South. Through this recruitment, three Black women contacted me. I interviewed two of them, and their stories have informed this book. The third woman ultimately chose not to share her story and did not disclose the reason for declining the opportunity. I have also drawn from several open access oral history interviews to learn and share, in the interviewees' own words, experiences that relate in some way to this project. In part, I consider this imbalance of white-to-nonwhite participants to reflect the disparity of raced experiences with unwed pregnancy in the United States in light of practices of hiding an unwed pregnancy, particularly through a residential stay at a maternity home. Revising my recruitment call to more explicitly invite participants with varied experiences with unwed pregnancy did little to aid in a more racially diverse set of interviewees.

Although I have worked to cultivate reciprocity and mutuality with participants, my need to depend on voluntary sharing has likely, and understandably, resulted in disparities related to who is compelled to respond and feel comfortable in sharing. While I worked to avoid—or at least rigorously trying to minimize—the easily extractive and thus colonial approach to research that can accompany participant engagement, my learning might be quite different if I had the capacity to employ a more long-term, relationship-cultivating, immersive participatory research design such as that modeled in Kathryn Edin and Maria Kefalas's *Promises I Can Keep: Why Poor Women Put Motherhood Before Marriage* (2005). More appropriate, I believe, would be for other researchers and/or activists who are members of or who have more organic or slowly cultivated relationships with communities not fully represented in this book to consider and explore other work on shame and/or reproductive experiences that people in those communities wish to discuss. I understand the potential benefit of such disparate inquiry approaches to align with the dynamism and inclusiveness of reproductive justice scholar-activists who "organize with people who think differently about issues or who focus on different issues but who agree to work together to achieve human rights goals" (Ross and Solinger 2017, 116).

In short, my intent is to draw from the wisdom of varied theoretical traditions to make a case for righteous reproduction as a manifestation of affectively steeped rhetorics of supremacy—a project that hopefully contributes in some way to the need for understanding and dismantling systems of oppression. I explicitly question how discourses about marginalized women who are pregnant and unmarried who have had experiences that reflect racist, ableist, and class-oriented white supremacist beliefs are deployed through rhetorics of shame. I examine this deployment in relation to public policy, shifting public discourses about young women's sexual and reproductive lives, and material manifestations of these discourses. I cannot account sufficiently for the felt experiences of non-white women in relation to shame. The first-hand accounts in this book are not meant to represent universal experiences, although some aspects of feeling ashamed likely are similar across contexts and embodied experiences.

The frame of righteous reproduction—one that is informed in large part by the open-endedness and dynamism of reproductive justice—enables me to make claims about the varied uses of this emotion and the interlocking (e.g., raced-, classed-, and age-based) implications of this use. I use this framing to bring together histories that are not often read together: namely, histories of what essentially amounts to revirginalization of mostly white women, histories of state-mandated reproductive violence, and histories of public considerations of causes and remedies of women's unsanctioned relationship to sex and pregnancy. As a book about supremacy, violence, and shame in relation to the recent history of unwed pregnancy, I cannot ignore race, despite my disinterest in perpetuating scholarly work that methodologically reduces Black lives, for instance, to being, in the words of Hartman, an "object of scholarly analysis" (Okeowo 2020). I cannot speak to all perspectives on this issue, and more important, it is not my place to do so. I am grateful to those women who have chosen to share their stories with me, and I hope that others will engage rhetorical examinations of shame that, in the words of Tarana Burke, enable an explicit "focus on Black humanity" or any other marginalized or multiply marginalized humanity (Burke and Brown, 2021, xi).

Enduring Shame traces stories—shared personally, published, extracted from media and archival accounts, or mostly erased and thus critically reimagined— circulating narratives, policy and juridical discourses, and the materially shaped spaces and processes of managing young women's pregnancy over roughly two decades to understand how experiences of being young and possibly or actually pregnant shifted during a period of feminist emergence, social and legal change, techno-medical discovery, and political and economy-oriented values in flux. Through the various periods and forms of change that function as the centerpiece of each of the following chapters, I focus on the rhetorics of shame that animate shifting deliberations and practices—even, and especially, when such shame is purported to have lessened in relation to such change. Across this historiographic examination, I argue that invocations of shame operate within a closed rhetorical system that fails to encourage new epistemologies or fresh and more just solutions to ongoing sites of discord. I conclude this book with a reflection on the need for more critical awareness of shame's presence in public discourses beyond the positive affordances of "writing shame" (Probyn 2010; Stenberg 2018) and in relation to the unjust effects of amplified uses of shame, namely call-out culture and cancel culture. I end by calling for more imaginative notions of how people can communicate in ways that operate beyond the pale of shame altogether—a challenging but potentially necessary task to take up in a contemporary moment when shame figures so centrally in public discussions and polarized debates about gender, power, and reproduction.

Studying the recent history of unwed pregnancy is relevant and useful work—not only in recovering stories that have been largely dismissed or, at minimum, insufficiently considered with respect to the expansive and inclusive possibilities of reproductive justice. Sexual shame persists, sexual shame permutates but rarely simply disappears, and sexual shame comes to bear on some of the most joyous, tragic, complex, and intimate aspects of people's lived experiences—historically and today. Sexual shame can influence one's sense of self and others—past, present, and future, yet shame (sexual or otherwise) functions as a deceptively powerful and misunderstood part of communication.

In his discussion of sexual shame, Michael Warner (1993) asks "what will we do with our shame?" and adds that "the usual response is: pin it on someone else" (3). *Enduring Shame* asks readers to appreciate shame's role in human communication and in relation to the recent history and ongoing struggles related to reproduction, pregnancy, and motherhood as fluid and vexed sites of identity and power. At a time of significant political and social unrest around reproductive sovereignty, legal protections, and the mass unsilencing of various forms of sexual violence, rhetorics of sexual shame are still largely misunderstood. It behooves those advocating for justice in these areas to revisit recent history to better understand the rhetorics of shame that linger today.

One

Unwed Pregnancy and Radial Rhetorics of Shame

Karen Wilson-Buterbaugh was a 16-year-old high school senior in 1965 when she became pregnant. As she shared with me in an email, she was taken out of school overnight and "whisked away" to a wage home in which she did chores and babysat children of strangers. In her seventh month of pregnancy, Wilson-Buterbaugh became a nonworking resident of a maternity home and then gave birth to a child that she would "surrender" for adoption. For a white woman, an unwed pregnancy was, in the time before, during, and even after the 1960s, a mark of incredible shame to be hidden and secreted at all cost; such women were given little if any plausible ability to resist a plan set in motion by parents, social workers, religious officials, and other authority figures coordinating on behalf of them and their "illegitimate" child. The plan resulted in a woman relinquishing her infant to a family who represented many things that the unwed mother was thought not to be: educated, capable, and deserving of a child. Often scared and isolated, these mothers had little choice but to acquiesce.

Wilson-Buterbaugh (n.d.) is one of many "invisible" women—estimates range from 1.5 million to 6 million in the United States—who temporarily hid an unwed pregnancy and then surrendered a child for adoption to keep that pregnancy a secret. In addition to losing a child, these women also surrendered their identity as mothers, obediently secreting their shamed past.[1] Fueling these practices was a desire for adoptable white babies that could be "gifted" to white two-parent homes. The typical euphemisms of relinquishment and adoption practices highlight the persuasive power of rhetorics of shame. "Giving" away a child could inaccurately suggest a self-motivated act on the part of the mother. The transactional language of the child as a "gift" (sometimes from God) subtly reinforced a belief among some adults that the child's birth was to be interpreted as a sign that it should be "given" to a childless couple. Such language runs counter to the feelings and perspectives of the once-unwed mothers I interviewed for this book.

My focus on rhetorical shaming highlights the gendered, raced, and classed aspects of this method for upholding righteous reproduction, since during this same era, non-white women's reproduction was differently engaged by majority white culture, for example, as an aspect of public health programs for curbing infant mortality or to limit non-white women's fertility through sterilization programs. When considered together, these experiences illuminate various violences enacted upon and erasures of young reproducing women. This chapter's story of shame primarily centers experiences of white and unmarried pregnant women who were implicated *because of their whiteness and class status* in radial rhetorics of private shame. Purity-based logics and corresponding rhetorics of shame were both well-understood and surreptitious factors contributing to white unwed mothers being exiled and put through elaborate charades of identity erasure. The ever-present yet elusive rhetorical quality of shame is what I attribute to several white interviewees telling me that their adopted children, with whom they have since reunited, cannot seem to understand the constraints under which they found themselves. This elusiveness, the relative absence of such stories, and these women's experiences as related to white supremacy culture and class status warrant this examination, particularly when differences in community expectations of unwed mothers and their children have been rationalized by the falsehood that only white children could be adopted.

Wilson-Buterbaugh contacted me after hearing about my research on unwed mothers. Wanting to share her story with me, she warned, "I would prefer not to work with anyone who will use the 'birthmother' term as we ARE the mothers of the children to whom we have given birth . . . not a label. We were labeled 'unwed mothers' during the Baby Scoop Era [a term that Wilson-Buterbaugh has coined]. I refuse to participate in the further oppression of mothers like me." As a feminist rhetorician, I consider it crucial to heed Wilson-Buterbaugh's wishes concerning terminology, but just as important, I wanted to hear more about how, for her—and, as I learned, some other mothers—the marker "birthmother" functions to extend oppression and silence. I asked Wilson-Buterbaugh for further clarification and she helped me to understand her position: "I used to use the 'birth' prefix early on, not understanding yet the negative power of it. Then I, and many others, evolved into using other ways to differentiate [ourselves] such as mother of loss, first mother, original mother, etc. It is an evolution. Some stay stuck in the 'birth' mode, sadly. Many, after learning what happened, the history of adoption practices and what their own personal experience was, even evolve into using 'mother of baby TAKEN by adoption.' Or even 'removed by adoption,' as they learned that they had no choice. No options presented."

Birth mother, as I have come to understand the term, is a label that directs attention to the unwed pregnant body as a site of gestation, a vessel for birthing a child that will not be one's own. In this historical context, it is a term that functions as synecdoche to deny an identity (mother) that was once, many years ago, erased.[2] Similarly, mothers commonly refer to the so-called "decision" to relinquish a child as "surrender," evoking the power wielded over them as new—but white, unwed, and thus largely disenfranchised—mothers and their feelings of having to submit to this unyielding authority.[3]

Undergirding the varied rhetorics of shame of this era are intertwined, private and public fears of moral failing (manifest in the "fall" of a virtuous and sexually pure white woman) as well as economic failing (manifest in a "fall" into state-dependency and/or poverty). These fears stoked the uses of shame and sustained its radial threat. At a 1963 gathering for one of the most prominent residential maternity home systems in the United States—the Florence Crittenton Association of America—one presenter's assessment of the state of unwed pregnancy reflects these interlaced fears. In "Unmarried Mothers, Immorality and the A.D.C. [Aid to Dependent Children]," the speaker proclaims that "Every day, year round, more than six hundred babies, unintended and unwanted, are delivered to their one parent—an unmarried mother. Of these six hundred babies, five hundred and twenty-five are lost to the public eye. They merge, publicly un-noticed, into the general population" (Perlman 1963). This alleged disappearance is explained as the effect of children being "absorbed into" the unwed mother's family, likely becoming the nominal child of the new grandmother, or the veiled process of "illegitimate" children being adopted into "legitimate" heterosexual, two-parent, economically secure families.

The presenter continues: "Many are *given* in adoption through solid social agency channels, to become the treasured and owned children of established families. Some are disposed of—*given* or sold—via black or grey market transactions" (emphasis added). Although the presenter notes that some women might be able to keep a child if, through the generosity of a family or sexual partner, the mother can manage to "resolve her conflicts or her precarious status," she concludes that the "remaining seventy-five of the daily crop of six hundred 'illegitimate' babies are carried by their mothers to the door of the public relief agency" (such as the A.D.C.). This assessment of the situation is telling because it accounts for the extent of this "problem," its various remedies, and the inconsistent ways that an unwed mother acts or is acted upon in relation to a pregnancy. It further champions the benefit of motherhood-erasing options that come at the expense of a pregnant woman in contrast to the least desirable option: a "crop" of "illegitimate" babies and their mothers who seek assistance at the expense of the wider public. Such remarks suggest that even among those in the role of providing aid, practices of secrecy, denial, and relinquishment in some form or another were a preferred way for an unmarried, white, and pregnant woman to navigate her shame, to contain its toxic spread among others, and to prevent its transfer to her child. In addition to invoking a fear of poverty and dependency, these ideas echo long-standing associations between ideal femininity and sexual purity as an antecedent to marriage and righteous motherhood—middle-class values that ensured that women could be (re)productive on behalf of the nation (Moslener 2015, 21–22).

In this chapter I question how a hiding and surrender mandate for white unwed women extended from gendered and supremacists logics, paying special attention to experiences of women who were unwed and pregnant during the 1960s. I theorize how rhetorical operations of shame manifested in and through such practices, and I consider the implications of these practices for women who enacted righteous image restoration through "going away." I use the term *going away*, then, in a capacious way—to evoke the constellation of interconnected practices that were specifically motivated by those upholding and/or ensnared in patriarchal and class-oriented, white supremacist logics of sexual purity as well as the related, radial affective and emotional intensities that accompanied these experiences. "Going away" as an act of profound secret-keeping and identity transformation necessitated persuasive discourses of humiliation that stripped women of their identities and primed them for processes of scapegoating and revirginalization.

Mapping various women's recollections of going away during the 1960s enables me to conceptualize radial rhetorics of shame by naming various apparatuses through which it was operationalized. Such shame rhetorics are *radial* because instead of only relating shame directed to or felt by an unwed mother, they reveal how shame was thought to have a viral or contagious quality. That is, shame in this case reflected a fear that shame could and would spread to those who remain identified with an unwed pregnant woman (parents, siblings, sexual partner, extended family, friends, community, others). Radial *rhetorics* of shame were varied (verbal, nonverbal, spatial, and so on) and encompassing so as to sequester the shame source and mitigate the contagion threat. Like the radial spokes of a tire, such shame moved between unwed mother and those who knew of "her" pregnancy, a figuration of possession that attached intercourse and its consequences to the one person in this case who was held culpable: the pregnant woman. Such movement reinforced an ecology of shame feelings and anxieties that help to explain the extraordinary hiding, silencing, lying, and secrecy practices I outline in this chapter. This rhetorical infrastructure culminated in identity relinquishment. Women were functionally revirginalized after the coordinated effort to hide and publicly erase any trace of pregnancy—a cruelly ironic and individuated aspect of this public secret. The radial shame operating at this time centralized white, unwed, pregnant women as the source of shame, but it activated a network of people, places, and activities—all connected to the unwed mother in question—that resulted in an encompassing shame culture meant to uphold righteous (read: white, normative, and marriage-contextual) reproduction. Such shaming stands in contradistinction from increasingly public interventions upon non-white reproducing women who were typically figured within dominant US culture as unrighteous because of their race or ethnicity and perceived (or actual) relationship to poverty.

The silences imposed and upheld by radial shame function paradoxically: as an attempt to conceal pregnant, unwed mothers (by removing them from sight), the act of hiding functions as part of an elaborate rhetorical performance that unwed mothers had to endure for the sake of those (parents, boyfriends, friends, others) who remained in public view, never openly acknowledging the reality at hand. In other words, girls went away to avoid shame, yet such hiding reinforced the notion that theirs was a shameful identity. The implications of these rhetorics of silence are not only physical or temporary, but rather enduring; they inaugurate a state of perpetual shame even though they are constructed upon the belief that women can and will forget their identities and experiences as unwed mothers. But as many such mothers have come to realize in their adult lives, the plan had a prominent flaw: the secrecy-through-relinquished identity it demanded. In this case, word of a "girl in trouble" often circulated as an open secret, and whispers gave voice to that which was never to be spoken. Whether "outed" or "outing" themselves or not, many such women still endure the weight of real and imposing secrets; they have borne the burden of an unarticulated social code that demanded they hold themselves singly culpable for a grave wrong (getting pregnant outside of marriage while being white) and that rendered them unfit to be mothers. When considered together, the following stories create a blueprint of attitudes, rhetorical messages, and rhetorical practices, all of which coalesced to enact radial rhetorics of private shame.

Listening to Stories of Marginalized Mothers

Although unwed pregnancy was considered shameful in the United States before the 1960s, this decade represents the apex of forced hiding and the near-mandate to surrender "illegitimate" white children for adoption. For many years, experiences of "going away" remained unspoken—shameful family secrets that could not be openly addressed, even by parents who tried to protect a daughter from social stigma that they found unfair. But in recent years, this silence has begun to break apart. Several authors—including Ann Fessler (2007), Rickie Solinger (2000), and Gabrielle Glaser (2020)—have produced monographs dedicated to examining practices related to unwed pregnancy in the United States. In addition (and sometimes as a result of such work), many mothers have ruptured imposed silences in order to talk to one another, share their stories publicly, and/or reunite with the children they surrendered for adoption. A few mothers have penned memoirs about how their experience as unwed mothers during the 1960s shaped their entire adult lives. Such historical scholarship and first-person accounts are critical contributions to recovering this portion of women's recent history—a history of women whose reproductive experiences are sites of marginalization, violence, systematic silencing, and degradation. These women's experiences relate to the reproductive justice concern for upholding safe and dignified contexts in which reproducing people can engage in the fundamental human right to have and parent children (Ross and Solinger 2017, 9). Additionally, this interrogation of rhetorics of shame contributing to constructed hierarchies of assumed racial and class-based difference supports the reproductive justice goal of understanding white supremacy as an ideology actively "used to promote unequal laws, practice, and social outcomes" related to reproductive lives (Ross et al. 2017, 17).

This gathering together of stories relies on published accounts as well as oral history interviews I conducted with twenty-seven mothers. These in-person interviews were part of several rounds of my institutionally reviewed and approved research program. Because women hid their unwed pregnancies anonymously, I relied on participant self-selection. I recruited in several cities in the Midwest, Eastern states, and South through newspaper advertisements and snowball sampling, or the processes of obtaining participants through word-of-mouth recruitment. All participants were women who experienced unwed pregnancy. Broadly commensurate with the demographic markers of women who hid an unwed pregnancy during the 1950s–1970s, all but three of these women were white. The purpose of these interviews was to listen to each woman's story of hiding and surrender and account for points of similarity across these narratives. Based on my inductive coding, I shaped this chapter from salient and overlapping aspects of these stories to investigate how once-unwed mothers frame their experiences as relating to shame and how their experiences during and after their pregnancy reflected orientations to and effects of shame. I follow interviewees' preferences for how they would like me to refer to them (by name or pseudonym of their choice) throughout the book.

Blending written and unwritten testimony supports my larger aim: to "honor and listen to the subjects of [my] research and respect the emotional and experiential context in which those subjects live and work" (Glenn 2018, 121). As historiographer Cheryl Glenn suggests, feminist rhetorical scholarship can "participate in a reciprocal cross-boundary exchange, in which we talk *with* and listen *to* others, to their vernaculars, experiences, and emotions" (122; emphasis in original). Drawing from published and unpublished stories allows me to tap into these experiences and emotions and to share the "vernaculars" of mothers who lived this history. By shedding light on a recent history that is still largely secreted and misunderstood, I interrogate sites of productive and unproductive silences (Glenn 2004) related to mothers' realities. I contextualize this history through archival and secondary research, although related sources rarely include the voices of women living this experience. Published accounts of mothers' experiences address hiding a pregnancy mostly as a precursor to longer and more detailed discussions of the experience of searching for and (sometimes) reuniting with a child surrendered for adoption. In practical terms, these publications do not illuminate the communicative acts that shaped women's experiences during and immediately after a pregnancy nor mothers' feelings and attitudes about these experiences.

I continue to incorporate published memoirs and interview excerpts into my scholarship because they provide additional information and because, in the case of memoirs, they reflect carefully crafted, sometimes researched, perspectives. All of these sources—the published and polished narratives, more improvisational and raw, if no less honest, interview comments, and those memoried texts in between[4]—that can shed light on secreted practices of the recent past. This mixed-methods and mixed-data approach extends feminist rhetorical practices that remain "in constant motion" (Schell 2010, 6–7) and feminist rhetorical historiographic commitments to resist closure (Glenn 1997, 174). Before turning to my analysis of these stories, I provide a brief contextual overview of the gendered, raced, and classed context of this era.

The 1960s: Sex and the Single Girl

The 1960s represent a time of instability and social change marked, in particular, by the civil rights movement, the fledgling women's rights movement, and a burgeoning gay liberation movement. Jackie recalled in her interview, "The change—the *pace* of change. It was so rapid in the '60s that it threw a lot of families for a loop. Women's rights, feminism, anti-war—the milieu was, it was just—it was anti-, anti-, anti-conservative parents." Empathizing with her parents' generation, she added, "Talk about having your back up against it!"

It can be tempting to reconstruct an era through its salient moments— instances of riot, of victory, and of death. But Jackie's sentiment is instructive in helping think about the pressures of the 1960s from the standpoint of families, and especially parents who held on to a moral conservatism that would not easily be diminished. The idea of the family figured prominently in discussions of international and domestic affairs in the post–World War II years; this preoccupation demonstrated a desire among many to exert some level of personal control in times of significant cultural change (Adams 1997, 21–22). Amid a chaotic social backdrop of, for instance, the abrupt and violent end of the fantasy of an American Camelot (with the assassination of President John F. Kennedy) and the pulsating bodies at Woodstock, many white Americans held tightly to the seemingly stable structure of the nuclear family and the fiction of its purity. The experiences of white and unmarried women reflect a concerted and elaborate effort to preserve and manage reproduction as a cornerstone of white privilege and upwardly mobile culture.

Reproduction in Non-White Communities

In the 1960s, non-white unwed pregnancy was also viewed unfavorably across communities, although it does not correlate with "going away" as described thus far. Historian Rickie Solinger contends that Black unwed and pregnant women "faced a forceful array of prejudices and policies" that threatened them and their children, even though in general, Black communities "organized" themselves to "accommodate" single mothers and children while the overwhelming response in white communities was to organize for the expulsion of the unwed mother (2000, 7). Those organizing efforts that were rationalized and operationalized by rhetorical uses of shame are the focus of this chapter. One complexity of this analysis, however, is the challenge of accounting for the internalized personal experiences and/or communal uptake of shame across communities and in light of these differences. In short, how did those in Black communities talk about pregnancy and its relationship to shame?

A relative lack of non-white women's accounts of their experiences (as I discussed in the introduction) prompts identifying other traces of this history. For instance, Suzan-Lori Parks's (2004) imaginative rendering of protagonist Billy Beede in her novel *Getting Mother's Body* reflects the dis-ease that this Black, unmarried, and pregnant character prompts in her 1960-era Texas town: "A girl with a baby-belly and no husband makes folks sweat" (50). While Billy's unwed pregnancy is a frequent source of tension among characters in this 2004 novel, the depiction of white unwed pregnancy in the 1956 novel *Peyton Place* suggests how communal feelings of fear and shame could manifest in expulsion of a pregnant person for the sake of the community's reputation. Rather than marking communal anxiety, the white unwed mother is othered in a way that immediately signals her defect and her disassociation with the community. "In Peyton Place there were three sources of scandal: suicide, murder and the impregnation of an unmarried girl" (Metalious 1956, 241). These fictional accounts are unsatisfying in their associative, unspecific affordances, even as they offer generalized truths about how unwed pregnancy was differently experienced *within* race-specific communities.

Additional historical traces provide details for further grappling with the varied relationships among unwed pregnant women, families and kinship networks, agencies attending to needs of unwed mothers-to-be, and the state. Saidiya Hartman has shared a family story of respectability, disclosing that her grandmother was rejected by her family—thrown out of the house—when becoming pregnant while at college. Berdie's child would be raised by Hartman's great-grandparents to save them from the shame of their unrighteous daughter (Okeowo 2020). Although Hartman does not date her story, it likely takes place well before the 1960s.

Reproductive justice scholar-activist Loretta Ross (2004–2005), however, has shared experiences as a Black, 15-year-old Texan who was raped by a family member and became pregnant in 1968. Ross's mother and a neighbor strategized what Ross should do, given her pregnancy. A promising student, Ross was being wooed by Ivy League colleges that were recruiting minority applicants, and she had already earned a scholarship to female-only Radcliffe College, the coordinate institution to then male-only Harvard University. The three ruled out Ross crossing the border to obtain a legal abortion—they were illegal in most of the United States at the time—since "too many women went to Mexico and didn't come back" (35). Instead, they determined that Ross should go to a Salvation Army home for unwed mothers. While Ross notes that this solution—having a baby in a "home," giving it up for adoption, and "com[ing] back and reintegrate[ing] into society"—was "pretty much the normal thing that girls did back then," she also notes that she was the only Black resident at her facility (35–36). At this point in history, such homes were responding to the mandate for hiding that emerged from white communities desperate to deny sexually active and unmarried—that is, unrighteous—daughters.

In terms of other experiences of non-white women, studies that reflect statewide trends are instructive. Mary S. Melcher's (2012) longitudinal overview of health policies and practices in Arizona during the twentieth century indicates that in rural areas of the state and on the Navajo reservation, public attention was given to high rates of infant mortality (107). Melcher amplifies the work of Dr. Pearl Mao Tang who became the chief of the Maricopa County Bureau of Maternal and Child Health in 1963, noting that Tang worked collaboratively with area leaders to lower the infant mortality rate in areas that also had comparatively high fertility rates (95). Tang and Navajo leader Annie Wauneka cultivated cross-cultural communication, established clinics in rural areas, improved health communication, and supported the creation of a mobile health clinic to reach rural areas (107–8). The focus here on health needs implies that unwed pregnancy was not a primary concern among non-white communities in Arizona during the 1960s. In urban Tucson, for example, a city that surely had a large white population, Planned Parenthood was distributing birth control to minors (those under 18 years of age) by 1969, encouraging parental consent but not demanding it.

At the same time, Indigenous families were being broken apart and young people relocated, part of a long history of forced acculturation by the

US government that would involve compulsory sterilization of Indigenous women—a topic I discuss in more detail in the next chapter. Covert population control programs funded by the Economic Opportunity Act of 1964 began affecting Indigenous women and represented localized implementation of President Lyndon Johnson's War on Poverty. Jean Whitehorse, a Navajo woman who was involuntarily sterilized in the early 1970s, has since shared her story of losing her ability to have children when receiving emergency (and non-reproduction-related) care at an Indian Health Service clinic. Whitehorse, who has only begun speaking out about her experience, admits thinking she was one of the only women who experienced involuntary sterilization even though the practice is now publicly recognized to have been deployed upon communities of poor women (Pember 2018, ¶ 18). Whitehorse has also helped to situate more fully her (and other Indigenous women's) experience with involuntary sterilization within the larger context of colonial practices of oppression and violence such as forced relocation, boarding school attendance, and mandatory assimilation into white culture (Tucker 2018). Though varied, these brief examples suggest that attention to unwed pregnancy as unrighteous, while a predominant aspect of white culture, was not necessarily a central reproductive focus in all communities. While shame related to unwed pregnancy may have been experienced across various communities and families within those communities, non-white people—for reasons of and sometimes beyond their choosing—were not as universally conscripted into pervasive white, patriarchal, middle class cultural beliefs about sexual shame.

Sterilization (euphemistically labeled *population control*) programs might have been funded by the US government but they were implemented at state and local levels, offering more opportunity to investigate how unwed pregnancy-as-problem manifested across different cultural and regional groups. For instance, a North Carolina-specific social services article published in 1965 outlines the long-standing debate around state-sanctioned and -funded sterilization of Black women on the basis of so-called illegitimate birth risks. The overview describes the first sterilization bill for illegitimacy in North Carolina (introduced in 1957) and discusses the subsequent work of researchers, advocates, and state legislators who contributed to debates about the state of "illegitimacy" among North Carolina's Black community and responses to this "problem" (Morrison 1965). Significantly, John R. Larkins, social worker and later state official, is described as developing a "North Carolina illegitimacy-prevention program" and spearheading fundraising efforts to construct a "maternity home for Negro unwed mothers" near Franklinton (7). The home, completed in 1964, figured into these discussions as an alternative to sterilization and as an opportunity for "self-help" within African American communities (7). Anti-sterilization efforts in the state were also construed by advocates as affording young Black women "the possibility of a happy married life" (8). This framing suggests the centrality of women's relationship to marriage and, therefore, that reproductive capabilities and rights remained in the context of marriage across white and Black communities—even when advocates for young women opposed state-organized and unjust sterilization programs.

In more general, national terms, unwed pregnancy and discussions of fertility control were increasingly linked to poverty and white people's fear of overpopulation, especially among poor, non-white portions of the population. Historian Kristin Luker (1997) argues that by the 1960s, and with a mass migration of Black people from the South to northern urban areas (like Chicago) in the wake of World War II, most Americans considered single motherhood to be a problem tied to poverty and race (54–56). The connection between race and income was not coincidental; because of long-standing governmental safety net programs that supported "respectable" mothers in need (especially those who were widowed and needed pension benefits) and that purposefully withheld support from "less respectable" mothers in need, a proportionately high number of Black single mothers lived in poverty by mid-century. As discourse about poverty in the United States assumed "a distinctly racial cast" (56), a focus on reproductive concerns among poor women was increasingly linked to fears of overpopulation and the threat of economic dependency. Luker explains that studies in the mid-1960s revealed that poor people (white and non-white) reported births that were unwanted, suggesting that contraceptive technologies were largely not reaching these communities (57).

Subsequently, a salient 1968 article by demographer Arthur Campbell stoked fears of a surfeit of fertility among the poor and especially those people who relied on public assistance (Luker 1997, 57). Campbell's argument bolstered support for intervening into poor communities with the goal of supporting fertility control and limiting births. According to Luker, the "troublesome solutions (such as involuntary sterilization) that, in an earlier era, had been associated with zealous pursuit of fitness [that is, a eugenics approach to averting feeblemindedness and other perceived forms of nonfitness] seemed much less relevant when it became clear that poor women were having children they themselves did not want" (57). By the time Campbell's article was published, Johnson's War on Poverty was well underway, including a "cautious" program for funding birth control for poor women.

In 1965, Daniel Moynihan, assistant secretary of labor in the Johnson administration, published a now-infamous report on a "new crisis in race relations" that, he argued, was fundamentally rooted in a bereft "family structure" among Black Americans. Drawing upon the argument that Black youth lacked "the socialization which only the family can provide" (Moynihan 2018, 48), the report reified notions that a two-parent family home is a safeguard against delinquency. It further pointed to "dominant" Black wives who were insufficiently subservient to husbands as a key reason for the failed African American family schema (30–31; 48). A call for intervention (by those white people in power), Moynihan's (1965) *Moynihan Report* marshaled fears of poverty, race, and population into an indictment of Black people and Black women, more specifically. Just two years later, the Grady Clinic, affiliated with Emory University in Atlanta, Georgia, started a protocol-less trial to test the effects of Depo-Provera, a long-acting contraceptive taken by injection. The eleven-year study, which started in 1967, was rife with violations of consent, faulty record-keeping, and poor communication with low-income subjects, many of whom were Black, who were experiencing a range of severe side-effects.

In sum, by the 1960s, and based on practices established primarily for white families/women as well as public interventions, non-white women were located by dominant culture as being outside the scope of white righteous reproduction, even if they, too, might have experienced sexual shame. In some instances health-based outreach was a nonmoral endeavor, in some cases Black communities sought to support Black women through an application of righteous standards, and in some cases medical interventions upon non-white reproducing bodies were linked to raced fears that linked purity-informed concepts of reproductive righteousness to state-level desires for population and economic control.

At the same time, some non-white women (such as Ross as well as one woman I interviewed who went to the Salvation Army home in Cleveland, Ohio) did use maternity home services. In both cases, these women's reflections on hiding and surrender demonstrate the desire for a more functional way of handling an unexpected pregnancy rather than their being compelled to perform revirginalized purity based primarily on the threat of radial shame. Wanda, a Black woman who had an unwed pregnancy in 1976 and who did not reside in a facility, shared that she did feel shame: "Shame. That was my name." Her story (to which I will return later in this book) reflects the reality of shame endured even when this shame did not culminate in an imperative to hide. Although the culture of "going away" was an artifact of a patriarchal and white supremacist pursuit of sexual purity, the radial effects of sexual shame did surely resonate within non-white families, kinship networks, and wider communities. Nevertheless, varied majority-led practices, majority-held attitudes, and sociological and economic theories of this time period set the stage for ensuing and coordinated sterilization abuses against non-white, poor, and/or "unfit" people. Such abuses were part of a wider landscape of reproductive politics and were indirectly justified as shoring up the sanctimony of the white family and the righteous reproduction it represented.

The White Family

Many white families at mid-century defined themselves around a concept of familial stability that linked consumerism with the performance of familial "normalcy." In the postwar years, middle-class, white families increasingly participated in a politics of respectability that established clear lines of in-group and out-group status. Performing this respectability, although not solely a matter of conspicuous consumption, nevertheless did involve owning specific products (e.g., cars, television sets) and creating domestic spaces enhanced by product purchases (e.g., kitchens equipped with modern appliances). These practices are part of a longer tradition of women's engagement with the market in an effort to display moral and domestic piety through consumption and the creation of a "tableau of female domesticity" that complemented the middle-class value of home ownership (Moslener 2015, 34–35). From a white picket fence to a perfectly set supper table, a "good" family could claim their status through visual and performative cues of "wholesomeness." Elaine Tyler May (2008) stresses that middle-class men and women "wholeheartedly and self-consciously attempted to *enact* cultural norms," and that by doing so they created and "reflected the standard against which nonconforming individuals were judged" (15; emphasis added). This standard was an intertwining of Christian notions of gendered morality and sexual purity and capitalist expressions of freedom of (consumer) choice and wealth accumulation.

The performance of such white, middle-class conformity was exemplified by popular television shows of the time. Such programming delivered an idealized reflection of the "normal" (read: white) American family—a construction that purposefully avoided controversy in order to attract viewers and appease commercial sponsors (Halliwell 2007, 158). Considering that television consumption averaged five hours per day per person by 1960 (Spigel 1992, 1) and that 60 million households owned a television by 1970 (Rielly 2003, 193), television programming surely influenced the way that many Americans gauged the boundaries of middle-class status. *Ozzie and Harriet*'s mundane, but "clean family normality" became the era's "reigning aesthetic" (Spigel 1992, 177). The Nelsons were a real family of actors and their depiction on television collapsed the dissonance between reality and fiction, the everyday and the ideal. The Nelsons, like the Cleavers (*Leave it to Beaver*), the Andersons (*Father Knows Best*), and the Stones (*The Donna Reed Show*), provided a model for domestic contentment, gender roles, and consumerism that American families could idealize and try to replicate. These families also articulated the proper flow of authority within the ideal nuclear family—from the wise father to the understanding, hyperdomesticated mother, down to the children. *The Donna Reed Show* featured the point of view of knowledgeable mother, Donna Stone, but her character's playful wit never realistically critiqued gender inequality. The title of *The Real McCoys* became popular shorthand for the authenticity of honoring the paternalistic family, and in several episodes, female characters' educational or entrepreneurial endeavors threatened to emasculate men in the family (Borelli 2012).

Simply put, in the milieu of the 1960s, many white Americans experienced uncertainty and aspired to attain the fantasy of gendered domestic hierarchy and conspicuous affluence modeled by the television families they encountered in their own living rooms. This programming is an important window into the visual politics of white kinship during the 1960s because of the visual and spatial rhetorics related to erasing white unwed mothers. How a family appeared—and the appearances of righteous familyhood as performed by seemingly innocuous television programs—was central to the story of raced and class-oriented righteous reproduction during this era.

These programs reinforced an ideology that sexism was good, natural, normal, and desirable. One subtext of the mid-century obsession with marriage was the belief that a woman's value was primarily measured by her sexual morality—in particular, that a girl should guard her sexual purity, dutifully and happily preserving her virginity for her future husband (even as men's sexual activity—a so-called "sowing of wild oats"—was seen, conversely, as evidence of virility and normalcy). The 1960s represent a time when this assumption started to come under scrutiny in various ways. "Theoretically, a 'nice' single woman has no sex life. What nonsense!" exclaimed Helen Gurley Brown in her 1962 best seller, *Sex and the Single Girl*. Brown's ode to premarital sex was, according to historian David Allyn (2001), "a wild confession, the kind of revelation that could destroy a woman's reputation, cost her her closest friends, wreck her marriage" (10). Brown, writing from a place of racial and economic privilege, gave voice to a then-radical notion of women's sexual freedom, which ostensibly was within their reach, given technological advances in the birth control pill and the intrauterine device (IUD). As is explained in greater detail in chapter 3, however, access to such birth control methods was impossible, or at least illegal, for many women—and unmarried women in particular because of this cult of purity.

By the later 1960s, a so-called sexual revolution was taking place in America, although this term was used flexibly to refer to a variety of countercultural expressions and actions including resistance to literary censorship and some nudity in theater and film. Nevertheless, "free love" became a principle and a practice for those who believed that the point of sex was to experience pleasure, and that sexual encounters could take place outside the confines of committed relationships (much less marriage). In theory, free love equated sex with freedom by using sex as a weapon through which to challenge a variety of establishment beliefs—religious, social, political, and so on. But in practice, free love simply did not "free" women, nor did it come without a price. It extended exploitation and domination of women even while purporting to free women from sexual norms. Calling out the leftist men who took advantage of this paradox, feminist liberationist Robin Morgan ([1970] 2000) proclaimed "Goodbye to All That" in her original manifesto of the same name, articulating that the "theory of free sexuality" was actually no more than male-directed sex on demand. Despite various social movements' attempts to identify, acknowledge, and rectify sites of injustice during the turbulent 1960s, the sexual double standard proved to be tenacious.

Normalcy, Scapegoating, and the Pursuit of Purity

Understanding white unwed pregnancy during the 1960s requires acknowledging that a woman's sexual purity was not simply her own. As memoirist Carol Schaefer (1991) explains, "You were a good girl or a bad girl, which meant you either went all the way or you didn't, no matter how long you were involved with someone" (7). Purity was an ideal that was ever so delicately tied to a white woman's reputation and, therefore, to what others said or did not say about her. A white woman's need to remain pure was intimately linked to her gendered role in relation to others in her life—her parents, siblings, friends, and others. A woman who was "loose" or "easy" was impure. Such terminology functioned as a code, communicating that a woman was rumored to have had sex or rumored to be willing to have sex. An "easy" woman's perceived impurity not only marked her, it also threatened the reputation of others around her. Because a daughter's sterling reputation was of such great importance, within the architecture of the family a good daughter was like a keystone, molded and positioned so as to secure the entire family's appearance of normalcy. The keystone's ornamental function pleases the eye while downplaying the function of the stone in ensuring structural integrity. Just as an imperfect center stone can compromise the strength and appearance of an arch, so too did a girl's reputation—which could turn from "good" to "bad" with one rumor—potentially imperil the entire family's image of decency (or, in other words, racial supremacy, middle-class status, and so on).

The constraining sexual norms that maintained a dichotomy between "good girls" and "bad girls" were felt acutely by those white women who became pregnant outside of wedlock. Recalling becoming pregnant as a sophomore in college, Schaefer (1991) "became like a child again" to her parents and agreed to hide in a home for unwed mothers (14). Although Schaefer did not feel like a "bad girl," the purity dichotomy continued to shape her thinking. She recalls imagining the others she will meet at the home, revealing the racial and class narrative she connected to the ideal of gendered sexual purity: "For sure they would be wearing tons of makeup, their eyes black and dramatically drawn like those of Egyptian harlots . . . Or else they would be dumb little country girls with used-up eyes and stringy dishwater blonde hair. Their boyfriends drove pickup trucks with rifles in the back widow and they probably weren't sure who the father of their baby was . . . Or maybe they would be motorcycle molls, with silver-studded black-leather maternity tops" (23–24). In fact, Schaefer actually encounters a house full of young (white) women much like herself: "It could have been our college cafeteria except for the big bellies" (24).

An obsession with normalcy resulted in a shared negligence in addressing the myriad reasons women—any women—became pregnant. Through my interviews, I learned that not all women who went away were teenagers, but a significant number of them were. For example, Mary, a resident in the Florence Crittenton Home of Toledo in 1969, specifically remembers two other residents: a 13-year-old girl who was sexually abused by her piano teacher at a lesson and a 14-year-old girl who had been raped by attackers when walking home from the library. Among those I interviewed, the youngest pregnancy was at age 14 and the oldest was at age 25. Overwhelmingly, the women who stayed at maternity homes said that the average age of girls in the home was mid to late teens. It is too easy for the term "unwed mother" to evoke the image of a young woman who has had consensual sex. Many women who experienced the trauma of stigmatized unwed motherhood as young girls, however, had little or no sexual experience. Some of these young women had not consented to sex, and some were naïve about the mechanics of sex in general and therefore were not even knowledgeable about what intercourse was or that they had experienced it. When memoirist Patti Hawn (2010) remembers the experience of visiting a doctor when her mother feared that she was pregnant, she recalls the incongruity of the doctor's questions about sex intercourse and her experience with her partner. "I hated those words," she admits. "That's nothing like what Robert and I had done" (118). In the words of Gayle, "we were children. You know, [at that moment] we are kids. This is probably the first thing we've ever done wrong." As these women soon discovered, a purity code allows no room for ignorance or error.

White babies conceived in the context of marriage symbolically functioned as outward, visible proof of the putative benefits of women's sexual purity: marital harmony, a (heterosexual) couple's sexual and emotional maturity and the resulting stability of this heteronormative gendered, familial order. Having a baby within marriage was not just a private choice but was also a promise to the community: by having this child, my husband and I accept the norms of this community and our gendered places within it (Adams 1997, 32). By understanding the inflexible codes of sexual behavior and the rhetorically saturated gender expectations of this era, one can start to appreciate the constraints bearing down on white unwed mothers-to-be. As Mary Jane, a resident staff member of one maternity home explained to me about the mostly young and well-educated women who came from across the United States to hide, "they were sure their family would disown them, and many would have."

The entire constellation of white cultural shame rhetorics operating in this context can be best understood as a rhetorical and physical practice of racialized scapegoating. A white daughter's precarious position in relationship to her family and loved ones set in motion elaborate plans of going away. Hiding was a performance (both literal and symbolic) that functioned as an act of atonement. As C. Allen Carter (1996) notes, to theorist Kenneth Burke, the scapegoat is "a process, not a thing" (20). One part of Burke's wide-ranging theory of language as symbolic action, the scapegoat process emerges from symbol-reliant society's inherent hierarchy, division, and desire for forms of perfection. Famously, Burke (1968) defines humans as "rotten" in their pursuit for purity (16). Frustration and anxiety with such a pursuit results in tensions that "must somehow be relieved," and thus humans "shore up" this disquiet and "seek someone to blame for [their] moral corruption, our social inadequacy" (Carter 1996, 18). In the 1960s, much added to white anxiety: waning assurances of the stability of marital conventions, racialized fears of people perceived to be poor and fertile, angst that raced codes of white women's respectability as unsexed girls or married mothers were being challenged, and a concern that the white nuclear family was being decentralized. At the same time, an adoption market for white babies would further enable the erasure of white unwed motherhood identities.

Although the notion of scapegoating suggests *disidentification*—a way to cast off the other, the nonself—Burke suggests that identification and consubstantiality (sharing substance with) are both central to the process of scapegoating. Specifically, Burke (1962) argues that scapegoating can only come from "an original state of merger, in that all iniquities are shared by both the iniquitous and their chosen vessel" (406). In other words, because persecutors see unfavorable characteristics of the scapegoat in themselves, the scapegoat is identified. Once that identification has been made (step one), there is a ritualistic alienation of the scapegoat, a division that separates the scapegoat (the daughter) from the persecutors (her family, in particular) and thus purifies them (step two). The scapegoating mechanism then rounds out by producing a "new principle of merger" in which the newly purified persecutors are unified, distinct from the persecuted (step three; 1962, 406). The scapegoat remains representative of the group, but the scapegoating process renders that person representative of "those infectious evils from which the group wants to be released" (Carter 1996, 18) and thus is able to transport said "evils" away from the group (Burke 1974, 39–40). The result is a ritualistic cleansing.

The belief that a white daughter becoming pregnant would bring humiliation onto her family is perhaps the most crucial aspect of the scapegoating process.[5] If the postwar family was a social fiction beholden to notions of racialized purity, the daughter's body becomes a canvas on which allegiance or deviance is expressed. Such a pursuit of purity relies on instances of impurity for definition (thus trafficking in a logic of boundaries and the possibility of body and spatial enclosure). Subsequently, *sexual impurity* functions as one form of "boundary pollution" (Douglas 1966, 155). The daughter *as daughter* is understood as a member of the family unit, and thus this familial context serves as the basis for Burke's initial step of merger, or identification. Because a white daughter's unwed pregnancy would have been a disgrace to her family, threatening to mark them as abnormal and impure, she was alienated to reestablish the family's purity. Scapegoating, then, as a form of symbolic and embodied action, enabled a woman's eventual return through performed revirginalization.

Expressions of Shame

As Lois explained to me when she recounted her story of doing "an unspeakable thing" by being pregnant outside of marriage, "they used shame on us." Lois's vague invocation of an agential "they" draws attention to rhetorics of shame that functioned to delimit white unwed mothers' options, suggesting that this shame was communicated by specific persons (e.g., parents, religious leaders, social workers) but also that it emanated from an indirect source: the racialized and socially held standard for white women's sexual purity. Lois's assertion that "[shame] is a powerful weapon, and they used it," illuminates that in the case of white unwed women during the 1960s, emotion was operationalized to indicate the severity of unwed pregnancy as a transgression against gendered expectations of righteous reproduction.

Shame also signaled that this was a transgression with severe ramifications, as I discuss below. Deborah, for instance, articulates how feeling ashamed was all-consuming and overpowering: "there was so much shame in that you are not good enough—you're not good enough to be a mother. And how would you—well, how dare you bring a baby into this? You know, there was no, there was no celebration of life—that this was a new life. It was, 'This is, this is a huge shame.' And I just felt that, well, um, they all knew better than I did, you know?" When considering once-unwed mothers' stories together, strategic uses *and* radial movements of weaponized shame become apparent. By mapping this moment of shame enveloping white unwed mothers-to-be, I add rhetorical nuance to Sara Ahmed's (2010) contention that shame is a "sticky" emotion that is communicated "atmospherical[ly]" (39–40). Although shame might have been experienced as an engulfing emotion to many unwed mothers at this time, attending to the specific moments that shame figures in their accounts enables a deconstruction and indexing of radial and communicated rhetorical expressions, practices, and spaces.

Communicating Shame upon Disclosure

Before white unwed mothers began to pack their bags, before they tried to figure out where to go to hide, they often had to let someone know about their pregnancy. A disclosure inaugurates the secrets yet to come; the flawed plan of denial is already compromised. The moments of awareness and disclosure— women finding out that they are pregnant and then sharing this information with others—is a salient portion of many stories of white unwed pregnancy in this era. And while a constellation of emotions (anger, disbelief, sadness) is part of mothers' recollections of disclosure, shame emerges as the predominant aspect of these stories.

Memories of disclosure illustrate the murkiness of intentionality's relationship to being shamed, as pregnant and unmarried white women felt the sting of shame directed to them even as they struggled to understand the state of pregnancy as an experience and exigence. For example, memoirist Margaret Moorman (1996) details an ignorance about getting/being pregnant that came up in various interviews I conducted: "When my breasts began to swell and ache, I told [my boyfriend Dan] I was afraid I had cancer. '*You are pregnant!*' he shouted. 'That is one of the signs!' Together we went to the telephone book, picked out the name of a gynecologist whose office was at some distance from our neighborhood, and made an appointment" (31–32). Once Moorman knew she could no longer deny her pregnancy, she informed her widowed mother that she and Dan were going to get married and have a baby. "My mother's reaction was instantaneous and explosive," Moorman writes. "'How could you DO this to me?' she shrieked" (39). Taking the response literally, Moorman admits that she "had not thought of her [mother] once, in fact, while achieving this remarkable feat of negligence and irresponsibility" (39). This reflection offers bittersweet, and instructive, humor; Moorman asks her readers to witness the incongruity of lacking the experience and perspective of an adult while having to account for her pregnancy.

As a legacy of the fallen-woman trope of decades earlier, white unwed mother status at mid-century was configured as an indication of an ontological shift, swift and decontextualized. As Pam explained to me, "the myth was that we were bad. You had sex and you got pregnant and that's, that's bad. I'm sure it wasn't only me, but I am the one who got caught." Yvonne's experience receiving "counseling" from a social worker also demonstrates this judgment of character: "The role [of a social worker] for the public was to counsel me about how horrible I was for becoming pregnant. I mean, back in those days, people would say 'You went and got yourself pregnant!' Like that's possible. It was a very, very common thing to say. . . . I really, truly felt that there was *nothing* I could have done worse, including killing someone coldheartedly . . . that could have possibly been any worse than getting pregnant and not being married. My parents never asked, [the social worker] never asked, the nuns at the maternity home never asked—no-one ever asked me anything about the relationship that led up to me being pregnant. It was just assumed that I was a slut and got pregnant." These shame messages quell empathy and foreclose opportunities for character restoration as a pregnant and unmarried person. They were communicated privately but function as indexes of a rigid, white purity code.

One key aspect of the radial qualities of communicated shame is how shame designated failure that refracted back onto the family. For example, Madeline remembers knowing that, once she became pregnant, she had "done the worst thing possible." Her mother emphasized this shameful state by telling Madeline, "'you're killing your father,'" attributing her and her husband's marital problems as well as the father's fear of losing his military job to Madeline's pregnancy (Fessler 2007, 239). This message that shame would boomerang back to the family is apparent in numerous interviews. Cynthia explains how this sense of contagion compounded feelings of isolation and alienation: "I was shaming the whole family; that was the outlook. I was shaming them. I told my boyfriend. He came to the house once. He told my mother that he would stick by me and help me financially—because we knew we weren't going to get married—help me financially and emotionally and a month later I called him and he had moved to North Carolina or something to be with his parents. So he was gone. I told my one girlfriend and she never called me again. So, that's my feeling. You tell people about this and they run away from you. So I never told my husband." For Cynthia, feeling ashamed set off a series of alienations and led to feelings of humiliation and the need to maintain a protective silence.

Similarly, Lois explained to me that her mother "came at [her]" when she learned of her pregnancy. Noting this extreme reaction with surprise, Lois continued: "[It was] like I just did something *to her.* She didn't have any concern for me; it was more punishment. And it was okay to do that back then. It was really okay [because] 'you disgraced this family.' [Speaking as her mother] 'Your father is going to lose his business.' [Speaking as herself again.] He was a businessman. A lot of people knew him." The fear of an unmarried daughter's perceived ability to draw shame on an entire family functions as the reason expressions of shame toward these women were so prevalent and intense. White unwed mothers were asked to see themselves as agents who were responsible for dire effects—both symbolic and material—that would implicate the entire family. This particular deployment of shame runs counter to what Ahmed (2004) refers to as *"the affective cost of not following the scripts of normative experience"* that functions as "a failure of myself to myself" (106–7; emphasis in original).

Rather than being shame that rests on and only on the unwed mother (a deployment of a sexual double standard), shame in these instances rhetorically resituates an individual's failure of the self so that it is understood to propagate, disseminate, and thus threaten the social and economic viability and interpersonal well-being of the family. Hall (2007) recalls the experience of receiving a radial expression of shame: "'You're pregnant, aren't you?' The words are hard, fierce. I cannot find my mother; she is gone, a million miles away, back in a place where there were no terrible surprises, where good girls don't draw shame on good mothers" (16). The reciprocity of such shame feelings is the primary way that the strain of a daughter's impurity was experienced within the family and communicated to her. Thus, this reciprocity serves as a marker of her relationship with others—a relationship that will eventually necessitate hiding and denial.

Rhetorical expressions of radial shame could be performed in other ways—more traumatic, more supportive, but in all cases reflective of the inescapability of the shame of unwed pregnancy in white culture. When 20-year-old Susan found out that she was pregnant in 1967, she was at a loss as to how to handle the situation. Unmarried and living at home with her parents, Susan remembers: "When I found out I was pregnant, I knew, number one, I could not tell my mother because I probably wouldn't live to see the next day. So, I just—I was a mess, I don't know, for a couple of weeks. Just trying to figure out what to do. I was going to run away. I was—I was just trying to figure out what I was going to do. And I couldn't *share* what was happening to me. There was no one to go to for help." Silenced, Susan decided to do "the only thing she could think to do," which was to tell her father about her pregnancy. Finding her father supportive, Susan nevertheless had to share this information with her mother. She remembers the day of this disclosure:

> Her gynecologist was the one I was going to. His office called her and said, "Harriet, we've noticed that you haven't been here for a while. Maybe you need to make an appointment." And so she did. So the doctor told mom and I was sitting out in the reception area and I heard her screaming all the way out to the reception area. And I was like, oh God, do I just get up and leave? What do I do? Well, the nurse came and got me and I went back there. And her reaction was so horrible. She called me a slut. She said, "Where did this happen?" She referred to his thing as a "big, hard," whatever her words were. I mean, it was devastating. It was beyond devastating. I felt like trash.

Susan's recollection centers on her mother's shaming discourse, which begins with an eruption of disappointment—a scream that pierced the professional space of the gynecologist's office. The scream inaugurates the shaming, and Susan's mother's revulsion is then amplified in her barrage of humiliating questions (which, I assume, took place in the consultation room, in front of the doctor, perhaps the nurse). Rhetorically, this performance functioned not only as communication to Susan, but also as an expression of shaming to be witnessed by those within earshot: It functioned as a semi-public performance of indignation. Such witnessed shame enables and deepens feelings of isolation and differentness on the part of the one shamed (Locke 2007, 148).

Describing a vastly different scenario, Faye remembers her moment of disclosure: "My dad, I don't know what he thought. I mean, [my parents] never, ever chastised me. Ever. They just never spoke about it at all. It was like it didn't exist." Perhaps Faye's parents embraced silence in order to cushion their white daughter from a pervasive shame culture to which they were complicit and over which they had no control. They may have struggled to find the right words in such a stifling culture of shame or may have felt fearful *and* loyal, a dissonance that rendered them mute. Both Susan's and Faye's recollections call attention to how shame's reach implicated mothers' families in ways they felt were inescapable. As these memories suggest, the presence of shame invokes the fear that an unwed mother's shame has already or will spread to those around her, making it not only communicated but also communicable.

Hiding as Embodied Rhetorical Performance

If moments of a white woman disclosing her unwed pregnancy were marked by painful expressions of shame, the stretch of time between learning of such a pregnancy and giving birth was overwhelmingly silent. This was a time of secret telling, secret keeping, and disappearing. As Lucy, a white woman who entered a maternity home in 1968 at age 14, explained to me, the "treatment [at the home] was not good. There were maybe sixty girls there. And we just bought it, with military precision. You know, no one said anything because you were trying to survive this and have a place to live." Yet Lucy also recalls the imbalance of this silence—the exceptions provided for those who *were* able to speak: "Everyday they'd say, you know: 'What do you have to give a baby? Do you have a job? Do you have a place to live?'" Not spaces for counseling and strategizing, maternity homes at this time were, instead, sites of disappearance that rhetorically confirmed white communities' desire for purging the imperfection of white unwed pregnancy. Even when residents were not posed such degrading questions such as those Lucy heard, they hid to assist the larger white community in recovering a visible semblance of social fitness through reproductive righteousness-as-normalcy.

"Going away" represents a semi-public performance of secreting that relied on anonymity, erasure, and physical spaces of hiding. Whether mothers relocated to a maternity home, wage home, or other residence in their own city or, for added anonymity, in another part of the country (a surprisingly common occurrence, especially because homes were frequently filled to capacity), hiding in some form was ubiquitous. Mothers' recollections of hiding suggest that these secrets functioned to stanch radial rhetorics of shame and thus operate as embodied rhetorical performances in their own right.

When Jackie became pregnant in 1965, she immediately felt the "shame, shame, shame" of unwed pregnancy. A white college student living away from home, Jackie nevertheless was still a daughter—still a reflection of her family. Jackie was raised in a religious household: her father served as an elder and her mother a deaconess in their church. If word got out that Jackie was pregnant, her parents believed, their family's social standing would be irreparably damaged. Her parents sent Jackie to live with her sister and her sister's husband in California until Jackie "began to show." This arrangement enabled the family to keep her pregnancy a secret until she could relocate to a home for unwed mothers. "That was the big thing—keeping it a secret," Jackie explained to me. "I don't think anyone knew except my aunt and uncle and my sister."

Keeping an unwed pregnancy a secret was so important, sometimes women kept the secret from those closest to them. Terri became pregnant in 1966, after having sex with her boyfriend of several months. Although he was her first and only sexual partner, Terri's boyfriend reacted to the news by doubting whether he was the father. The boyfriend returned to college, leaving Terri behind. "Anytime I tried to call him after that," Terri explains, "those were the days when you had to use money in the phone and I was in a highway phone booth. And he would just take his time and not come to the phone and I would use up all my change. And I never heard from him again." Because Terri was "alone and pregnant" and because her (white) family was "very strict," she decided to keep her pregnancy a secret from them, instead making up a lie that she was joining the Peace Corps. "And I was scheduled to go in and like two days before I was scheduled to leave, Catholic Charities called my home thinking [my parents] already knew. And that's how my mother and father found out. No one else in the family ever knew."

Various networks of maternity homes—especially those run through agencies like the Florence Crittenton Association, the Salvation Army, and Catholic Charities—offered a "private" space dedicated to this business of hiding. But not all women did—or could—hide in such facilities. For example, when Barbara, who is white, became pregnant in 1966, her family decided that she should stay at home: "I wasn't sent away, although my mother told me about those places. But I was hidden away at home. I had a bedroom up in the attic. We had a bedroom up there; it wasn't like they made one and just put me up there like a squirrel. But, you know, whenever the doorbell rang I had to run upstairs. I couldn't be seen. I had just disappeared." Barbara's experience illustrates the extent to which hiding was a central feature of "going away," even outside of the infrastructure of maternity homes.

Sandy had a different arrangement for upholding the secret of a white, unwed pregnancy. She and her high school sweetheart were planning to get married before she became pregnant in 1967. Despite this promise, Sandy's boyfriend, who was away at college, began to distance himself from her when she told him of her pregnancy. Traveling from New Jersey to North Carolina to be with him, Sandy was planning on applying for admission to a Salvation Army home but realized that staying in a motel was cheaper and thus a wiser choice, since she needed to rely on her personal savings to stay hidden through the pregnancy. "While I was in the motel, it was just me. And I did consider suicide and had my note all written," Sandy remembers. Her boyfriend had, by this time, begun dating someone new, although he did not admit as much to Sandy or his parents, who already considered Sandy part of the family. Pushing aside her feelings of desolation, Sandy remained at the hotel until the very end of her pregnancy when she went to a maternity home. She kept the secret of her pregnancy from everyone until she could no longer hide the information with the man and woman who were to have been her in-laws: "They were very nice. I say they were very nice because in that day and age, my parents didn't know—nobody knew—just he and I. But I knew that I had to do what I had to do because of how society was. So, um, so I promised them, 'Don't worry, nobody will know. I won't tell anybody.' And I knew that they couldn't let their neighbors know because if—God forbid—the neighbors knew! And his three sisters didn't know."

For Sandy, hiding was a necessary responsibility, one that she bore alone, tragically, on behalf of her family as well as people who would be socially injured by their association to her. In this way, hiding also functioned preventatively. It preempted the shame families feared they would experience by proxy if a daughter's situation became public knowledge—a threat that reflects the *sociality* of shame as an emotion that signals feelings of being revealed to or seen by others, even when not in their actual presence. Yvonne remembers, "I was not even allowed to visit [my parents] on a Sunday [once I was living in a maternity home]. Because that means I'd have to go to church with them. And what if somebody saw me? What if somebody saw me and knew that I was pregnant? Well, I didn't look pregnant, but that didn't matter."

Shame, as an experienced emotion, "feels like an exposure" (Ahmed 2004, 103) and thus typically moves the ashamed to look down, slump, or fold into themselves. These bodily responses are an effort to take up less space and make oneself smaller. The practice of secreting and hiding an unwed mother, then, can be situated as an extreme—and indefensible—manifestation of this embodied shame performance. Experiencing the fullness of this erasure, memoirist

Julie Mannix von Zerneck describes the month she spent in a "first-class sani-torium" and then her longer stay in a "state hospital" (i.e., a residential facility for those with mental illness) in 1963 (Mannix von Zerneck and Hatfield 2013, 91). Unaware at first that her mother arranged the stay at the state hospital under the pretext of her daughter's suicidal tendencies—a move that might have made her, a white woman, eligible for an approved abortion—Mannix von Zerneck recounts the experience of being assessed by a hospital staff member. Not receiving any response to her pleas for help and insistence that she did not belong in such a facility, Mannix von Zerneck shares that subsequently, she "refused to utter a single word. I silently retreated inside myself—a condition that is, I would later find out, called *elective mutism*" (13; emphasis in original). Reflecting on this response, Mannix von Zerneck contends that "refusing to talk had given me a sense of control where I had none before. I found great power behind my unspoken words" (91). This recollection suggests that elective silence was commensurate with the erasure of presence and identity that a rhetorical performance of hiding signified.

Hiding as an embodied act also functioned in ways that are notably para-doxical—both obscuring and revealing unwed pregnancy. Even though many women with whom I spoke assured me that family members never knew about their pregnancy, the open secrets of young white women "needing" to hide and finding ways to do so suggests that this concealment was not foolproof. Secrets in the service of silence can still be spoken, even in hushed voices. As Schaefer (1991) remembers, "Out-of-wedlock pregnancies were an intriguing topic of conversation, but never discussed except in whispers and innuendoes" (17). One mother, also white, recounted to me the stunning effect of having a classmate casually ask, "What did you have?" when she returned to high school. Not knowing how to answer this question about the sex of her baby, the mother remained silent. "I backed totally away," she recalls. The secrets and lies related to hiding could not render mothers impervious to attention, even if they were pulled from public view as soon as an unwed pregnancy was confirmed or in some cases merely suspected. The juxtaposition of, on one hand, practices of hiding and erasure and, on the other, the common knowledge of the social expectation and ubiquity of secret-keeping underscores the artifice of this ar-rangement. It also emphasizes the familial and social sacrifice mothers person-ally made for the fiction of "honorable" sexual purity.

Some women who were compelled to hide were nevertheless encouraged to reckon in paradoxical ways with their "sin." When Yvonne became pregnant in 1967, her parents arranged for her to have regular meetings with a social worker, a woman who consistently discouraged her from imagining the possi-bility of keeping her child. While presumably the role of the social worker was "to counsel me, I guess," this woman wanted Yvonne to graphically recall her sexual encounter. Yvonne remembers that during one of the sessions, the social worker asked her whether she enjoyed "it," a comment that initially caught Yvonne by surprise. "She's asking me if I enjoyed sex!" she remembers. "We're Catholics here, aren't we? We don't talk about this stuff! It was just really, really, really, really creepy that she asked me that. Shockingly creepy."

While Yvonne's surprise and repulsion eclipsed memories of feeling shame in relation to this question, understanding it within the context of the role of the social worker demonstrates that more than just being disturbing, the question functioned for Yvonne as an experienced amplification of shame. Instead of counseling or deliberating on Yvonne's options as an unwed mother, the meetings were a space for recycling shame, ensnaring Yvonne within an invasive, surveilled shaming loop that indirectly rationalized the coordinated intervention into her life as a pregnant woman and justified a pseudo-public management of her fertility. Wilson-Buterbaugh (2017) writes of a similar experience in which a social worker who "never discussed keeping my baby or discussed any rights I might have had at this time" instead was "more interested in my sexual experience" (26). Like Yvonne, Wilson-Buterbaugh recollects how these exchanges were "extremely awkward" (26). In both cases, this coercive reactivation of shame highlights institutional exploitation of power to repeatedly punish a mother by providing a witnessing audience to "her" transgression even as she was hiding as a means of embodied denial and invisibility.

Yvonne also shared with me memories of receiving a letter from her 14-year-old sister that explained how "dreadful" Yvonne was. Yvonne's sister also described her shame being discussed "around the dinner table *and* the supper table *and* the breakfast table" because she was a "slut" and a "whore" who had "ruined the family name." These epithets emphasize Yvonne's deviancy through allegations of hypersexuality. Many mothers explained to me that to be white, unwed, and pregnant elicited accusations of being a "slut" or "whore" even when there was no evidence of a woman having had multiple sexual encounters. Yvonne was devastated by the letter but did not hold her sister accountable; she knew that the talk of her sexual impurity came from her parents and that her sister just absorbed, and regurgitated, this shaming language. Yvonne recognizes the ritualistic quality of her sister's shame, and she finds solace in distinguishing between her sister's rhetorical performance and what she imagines to be her sister's true feelings. Such rhetorical engagement with taboo is not unique; Michele L. Hammers (2006) argues that when the sexual female body is effaced from public view and discourse, it garners attention for paradoxically residing at the "border of amplification and erasure" (227). In this instance, however, the publicity of shaming—here within the family— underscores the threat of contagion that a white woman's sexual transgression prompted and the role that an unrighteous daughter could privately play in reinforcing the strictures of gendered sexual purity.

The "Home" as a Spatial Rhetorical Response

Most of the women with whom I spoke spent at least some time at a maternity home before delivering their child. Such homes were a typical feature of hiding and secret-keeping practices, represented by facilities run by the Florence Crittenton Association, the Salvation Army, Catholic Charities, and various other independent agencies. As a highly coordinated response to unwed pregnancy, such homes function rhetorically in two ways. To the larger community, homes for unwed mothers served a spatio-rhetorical role in assuring that white unwed pregnancy would remain intolerable and invisible. To the women who resided in the homes, these spaces fostered emotionless regimentation and muted, anonymous domesticity. In this way the spaces were suasive because they primed unwed mothers to relinquish their mother identity as they relinquished their child for adoption.

Spatial rhetorics functioned in particular ways that could be "read" by those outside the home. Schaefer (1991) recalls wondering about maternity homes before she became a resident at one. She ponders whether "parents drove by and said a silent prayer to spare their daughters and themselves that pain and humiliation. Or said a prayer out loud in thanksgiving that their kids had made it through and were well on their way to fulfilling their parents' dreams" (21). The outward function of the maternity home was to reassure nonresidents of the presence of a space for corralling, enclosing, and visibly hiding white unwed pregnant bodies. Here the rhetorical functions of these structures relate to their "existence" and how that presence exerts a spatio-rhetorical "suasive" form (Enoch 2019, 123). Like the World War II-era childcare centers that Jessica Enoch has studied, maternity homes as architectural spaces "announced their availability and support" to the wider community (135–36). Enoch argues that childcare centers were strategically located and constructed to communicate "relief" and foster trust in the services that were likely to raise doubts among working mothers (136). Similarly, maternity homes provided succor to white families keen on visibly upholding purity standards while potentially instilling fear and disidentification among their residents.

Being privately run facilities, maternity homes of the 1960s did not exude an institutional or sterile feel. Homes were mansions (e.g., those long-owned by the Florence Crittenton Mission, in existence since the late 1800s), cottages, or more contemporary, institutional buildings nevertheless designed to feel homelike. According to the mothers I interviewed, homes were typically in a well-travelled part of town, although those in suburban areas generally had a privacy fence surrounding the property. In her history of unwed pregnancy in the United States, Solinger (2000) describes "the world of maternity homes in postwar America" as "a gothic attic obscured from the community by the closed curtains of gentility and high spiked fences" (103). As "material formations" (Enoch 2019, 135), such conspicuous, often looming, structures persuaded communities to be aware of their presence and their civic function in maintaining the appearance of righteous reproduction.

No matter the façade of each facility, the language of "home" was pervasive across the various agencies providing services to unwed mothers. By creating physical places that (to varying degrees) *looked* like private residences and by deeming these various buildings each a "home," the social service and religious agencies running the homes constructed a particular spatiality. *Spatiality* connotes that space is not neutral, empty, or fixed, but rather a "relational *social product*" that can be altered, used, and experienced in various ways (Nunley 2011, 40; emphasis in original). Spatiality and the related concept of *practiced spatiality* rely on the notion that "the conception, understanding, habitation, and use of the materiality of space and place mediate the encounter through power and ideology" and that place can be usefully interrogated for its connection to the practices of bodies within it (40–43). The spatiality of these homes suggested a domestic site of femininity while residents remained aware of their status as unrighteous women needing sanctuary and protection.

It is impossible to account for how the spatiality of a variety of maternity homes was experienced by residents; nevertheless, it is plausible to suggest that the homelike environment was created to foster a sense of familiarity and comfort for these women. But "home" has also functioned as an enduring symbol of women's "proper" place—an environment in which they could cultivate "true womanhood" ideals such as submissiveness, domesticity, purity, and piety (Welter 1966, 152). Thus, the spatiality of maternity homes likely reminded residents of mid-century gendered values and allowed residents to cultivate domesticity (through the habit of performing household chores, for example). More than being just a place for "biding time" until delivery, the spatiality of the homes likely reinforced the supposed link between white womanhood, domesticity, and righteous reproduction. Although such spatial meaning would have been subtle, feminist geographer Linda McDowell (1999) argues that spatiality is, in fact, highly persuasive. "Spaces exercise heuristic power over their inhabitants and spectators by forcing them to change . . . their behavior," according to McDowell, "and sometimes, their view of themselves" (25). Interviewees often referred to a home as a social space, similar to a closed sorority house, where men were generally not permitted entrance. Despite this spatial division between outside and inside, however, these women did not report bonding or sharing a sense of identification with one another.

Despite what maternity homes communicated through spatial rhetorics to the larger community, they could have different meanings for the residents who stayed in them. Audrey, a white woman I interviewed about her stay at a home in 1970, emphasized that it represented literal imprisonment to her—a sentiment that nearly parallels that which Ross recalls from her time in Texas. Audrey described the structure as a big, brick mansion built in the early 1900s, noting its dark façade and the 8-foot high, wrought iron spiked fence that encircled the property. Although Audrey's memories of the house itself evoked the containment she experienced while there, she acknowledges that it was nevertheless a "gorgeous home" that had probably once been a private residence for a captain of industry. Jackie, who lived at a home in Cleveland in 1965 more openly acknowledged the opulence of that house. Describing this home as a "gorgeous, huge old white elephant" on "millionaire's row," Jackie suggests the saturation of meaning that these homes had accrued by the middle of the twentieth century. Houses congratulated a community for its benevolence on behalf of "bad girls," shrouded these women while communicating the "need" for hiding, and loomed, hulking and silent, to women who entered their doors and surrendered voice, autonomy, and—in too many cases—the acknowledgement of their own motherhood.

In *Wake Up Little Susie,* Solinger (2000) provides an overview of the ways in which community members came into contact with maternity homes. For instance, even though homes charged a fee for entry, many mothers relied on community chest support and the help of volunteers and boards of directors who could fundraise on their behalf. Solinger argues that, overall, communities found the presence of maternity homes "repugnant" (126). I counter that communities found unwed *mothers* repugnant but maintained a grotesque fascination with the ideas of the homes themselves, which prompted elaborate, though ineffectual, efforts at keeping unwed pregnancy a secret (such as atypical architectural preservation, the construction of high fences, and the circulation of the anonymizing images such as those included in this chapter).[6] By the middle of the century, homes for unwed mothers performed a polysemous spatiality that played a significant role in the cultural narrative that "going away" and "forgetting" was the best response—the only response, as suggested to their residents—to white girls who "got themselves" in trouble.

Materials marketing maternity homes by mid-century emphasize these homes as privatized sites of domesticity that reify the notion that this type of "home" is a highly feminized space that replicates other group living arrangements for women (fig. 2). Emphasis on sleeping and eating quarters promote domestic order and tidiness. Materials evoke the typical rhythms of daily life, and images of a private "homelike atmosphere" do not call attention to needs of pregnant women, even as captions mention "a medical program" and the availability of "psychiatric services." By overwriting the home's primary function of hiding so-called illegitimate pregnancies with the normalcy of domesticity, such materials suggest that these spaces invited female identification *inscribed* by patriarchal power, even as they functioned as spaces for being pregnant and waiting to give birth. The coded space of feminine domesticity that makes these spaces appealing in a brochure obscure the patriarchal and power-driven reasons for their existence and their performance *as* a home-like space. Feminist geographer Nancy Duncan (1996) argues that historically, the personal freedoms of the head of the household—usually a male—have tended to delimit and sometimes deny the "rights, autonomy and safety of women and children who also occupy those spaces." Thus, such homes are spatial expressions of the confluence of privacy, masculinity, male autonomy, and property ownership. In short, argues Duncan, "as a relatively unregulated sphere the private is a place where men have traditionally dominated their families and the privacy to do so has been jealously protected" (131). Thus, symbolically, the home was the haven of femininity, but in practice, the power wielded inside the home pivoted on the fulcrum of male power and dominance.

Within homes, spatial rhetorics held sway for residents in differing and varied ways. For some, the home functioned as a safe haven, a place where, as Faye remembers, she could finally take off the girdle she had been wearing to hide her belly and just *be* pregnant. Yvonne remembers that in comparison to meeting with her social worker, who always asked, "What makes you think you have *anything* to offer [a baby]?" the home was a relief because "there, no-one was saying those things to me." For Jackie, staying at a home was itself neither good nor bad: it was merely "putting in time," a means to what would be a very difficult end in many cases. Yet Nancy Ann's experience at a Catholic Charities home was traumatizing. She writes, "I compare my stay there to anyone who is abducted by a cult. I was brainwashed with propaganda of how sinful I was. I was treated like a second-class citizen who deserved to be treated as such for my sins and given tasks to do that no one nine months pregnant should be allowed to do, such as working in a laundry where the temperature exceeded 100 degrees. All of this was referred to as my punishment" (quoted in Wilson-Buterbaugh 2017, 73). It can be challenging to make sense of the rhetorics of and in these spaces when experiences varied so significantly. In addition to bearing witness to these differing lived realities and recollections, one more encompassing reality can be drawn. Even when not punitive, the space of the maternity home—as a material construction and a place filled with meanings, associations, and types of use—functioned consistently to dissuade residents from seeing themselves as mothers-to-be.

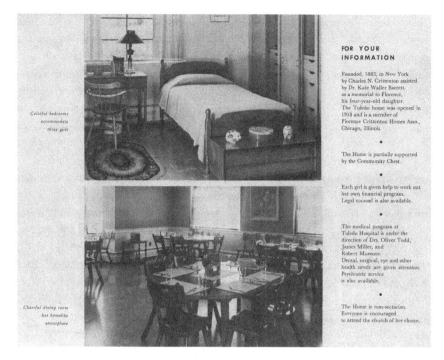

Colorful bedrooms accommodate three girls

Cheerful dining room has homelike atmosphere

FOR YOUR
INFORMATION

Founded, 1883, in New York
by Charles N. Crittenton assisted
by Dr. Kate Waller Barrett,
as a memorial to Florence,
his four-year-old daughter.
The Toledo home was opened in
1918 and is a member of
Florence Crittenton Homes Assn.,
Chicago, Illinois.

•

The Home is partially supported
by the Community Chest.

•

Each girl is given help to work out
her own financial program.
Legal counsel is also available.

•

The medical program at
Toledo Hospital is under the
direction of Drs. Oliver Todd,
James Miller, and
Robert Muenzer.
Dental, surgical, eye and other
health needs are given attention.
Psychiatric service
is also available.

•

The Home is non-sectarian.
Everyone is encouraged
to attend the church of her choice.

Figure 2. The interior of the Toledo, Ohio, Florence Crittenton Home, ca. 1955–60.
Social Welfare History Archives, Florence Crittenton Collection, box 23,
folder 5, University of Minnesota Libraries.

Understanding how maternity homes imagined their own services is challenging given the vast number of facilities and variations among them, although some general conclusions prove instructive. Preserved in various Florence Crittenton Association archives are a variety of rule books—handmade documents meant to introduce new residents to the home and acquaint them with expectations. A circa 1960 book from the Toledo, Ohio Florence Crittenton Home welcomes new residents by assuring that "This is your home now and we want you to feel welcome right away. We're proud of it—we hope you will be too." The note continues by suggesting, indirectly, that residence in the home offers more than just a place to hide: "Let living here be an experience that helps you prepare for the future, when you will have your own home or some other interesting career, and be better able to master the daily problems of living and getting along with others. You will be with us until three weeks after delivery; you can make each day count. Think, as you read the following pages, for upon your acceptance of our ideas depends the usefulness of this booklet" (*Guide*

Book n.d.). A variety of similar books, distributed at other Crittenton homes, communicated the same message: the home was a route to rehabilitation and reinvention—a place where an unwed mother could create a better version of herself. This aspect of the persuasive function of the homes is one to which I return in the conclusion of this book, as I describe the organization's reconfigured, now justice-oriented, and sustained support of marginalized women outside the constraints of this era, one marked by racialized, class-based demands for physical hiding and identity erasure.

Overwhelmingly, the women with whom I spoke did not remember the maternity homes as draconian in the way that Nancy Ann, Audrey, and Ross did, although in almost all cases they were highly regimented. Katherine explained that days were routine: everyone took meals together and did regular chores and laundry. Most women remember being weighed daily, seeing a physician regularly, and doing group exercises in the home to stay fit. Nearly all the women remembered there being a great deal of "free" time, during which they watched television, read, crocheted, and talked. Many of the homes offered religious services: in some, attendance was required and in others it was optional. At some homes, women were allowed to leave the facility if they signed in and out and followed curfew; other homes were far more restrictive about women remaining inside the home or at least within a fenced yard. Most generally, however, the rules of the home kept it running smoothly more than they disciplined the residents. As Deborah explained to me, "I don't remember anything being written down . . . there wasn't a lot of rebellion. It was like, you had to follow the rules. Because what was going to happen if you were thrown out of here? Where were you going to go then?"

One of the few restrictions that was exercised with some regularity was a code of anonymity. Many residents were instructed to change their name entirely or refrain from using their last name. Nancy Ann remembers that her "clothes were taken away," her "name was changed," and she "was not able to connect with the outside world" (quoted in Wilson Buterbaugh 2017, 73). As Gayle explained, "You weren't supposed to talk specifically about where you came from, but we all did. They tried hard to make it confidential." From within the homes, some residents befriended one another and shared their stories, violating the code of secrecy.

The visual rhetoric produced by and relating to maternity homes emphasized this desire for strict anonymity. Brochures and news articles consistently portrayed an indistinguishable unwed mother on the front steps or inside the maternity home—but always facing away from the camera (fig. 3). As a visual argument, such images persuaded viewers to believe that the anonymity could be and was upheld, even when in so many cases, it was not honored. The insistence on anonymity within the homes both functioned to protect unwed mothers from shame and reify the notion that being an unwed mother was shameful (fig. 4).

Mothers-as-residents, despite their proximity to one another, overwhelmingly did not share feelings of anger and injustice or desires to resist the denial of motherhood (even if some did, significantly, use their agency to surreptitiously resist rules of anonymity). Maternity homes cultivated emotionless regimentation and muted, anonymous domesticity. This aspect of the homes' spatiality stands in stark contrast with that of other feminine-coded and pseudo-domestic spaces such as sorority houses, which Charlotte Hogg (2018) suggests contribute to "pervasive" rhetorical messages of the "work of belonging" for young women joining a Greek organization (424–25). The homes' spatial invocation of domesticated white womanhood and its related sexual purity as well as the practiced spatiality of a future self that will deny unwed motherhood all materialize the timelessness of radiating shame. Ahmed (2004) contends that for shame to be restorative, that is, for one to be restored from and by shame, it must be "seen as temporary" (107). Maternity homes did not spatially afford residents an ability to collectively or individually work through public scripts of sexual shame, and in this way they served as suspended spaces of atmospheric

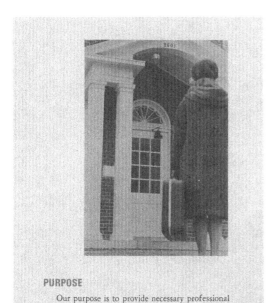

Figure 3. Brochure for the Topeka, Kansas, Crittenton Home, ca. 1958–61. Social Welfare History Archives, Florence Crittenton Collection, box 22, folder 5, University of Minnesota Libraries.

PURPOSE

Our purpose is to provide necessary professional services to the unmarried mother in a friendly helpful atmosphere so that she may have real opportunity for personal development and for making sound plans for herself and her baby.

HOME LIFE

Girls at the Home and staff members cooperate to maintain a pleasant, home-like environment at Crittenton. The Home is attractively furnished and well-managed, with emphasis on its liveability and comfort. In this carefully-supervised group life, each girl can acquire a sense of "belonging" and the ability to adjust to problems and other personalities. Training in homemaking arts, personal grooming, and good health habits is given each girl. Individual responsibilities for household tasks are determined by each girl's preference and physical condition.

BACKGROUND

Efforts to aid unmarried, pregnant young women in Chattanooga began in 1877 by a group known as the Woman's Mission Home Board, which in 1897 became affiliated with the national Florence Crittenton chain. Today our Home is one of 54 homes operating throughout the United States under the guidance of the Florence Crittenton Homes Association.

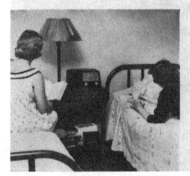

Figure 4. Image of "home life" from a Chattanooga, Tennessee, Crittenton brochure, 1950s. Social Welfare History Archives, Florence Crittenton Collection, box 24, folder 5, University of Minnesota Libraries.

shaming that perpetuated for mothers their "inhabitance of the 'non'" (107). Further, as familiar-looking spaces of emotionally coercive protection—rather than that of belonging or therapeutic reckonings with feeling—a maternity home primarily served the needs of families (and collectively, white normative publics) threatened by radial, radiating shame. The inner spaces of maternity homes—the spaces where mothers waited as childbirth neared—were, then, shame-infused places that stymied women's understanding and recognition of themselves as mothers, furtively priming their pregnant residents for the forgetting that they were told would come with child relinquishment.

Nowhere Left to Hide: Punishing Labor and the Birth of Loss

The secrets and erasure of hiding functioned as a precursor to the final and, arguably, the most painful iteration of radial shame. Unwed mothers passed weeks, even months, in hiding, but the adults coordinating this hiding generally neglected to inform the mothers of what would happen during labor and delivery and after the birth of their child. Thus, the silences surrounding the birthing process enabled degrading, often disciplining, medical approaches that symbolically and physically divested these mothers of agency over their own labor and delivery. In the days after delivery, when mothers should have legally been able to decide whether to consent to an adoption, many women were physically barred from seeing or holding their children, enduring even more shame and isolation. Silenced (or coerced or extorted, as in the case of Yvonne who was reluctantly given the "choice" of keeping her baby upon payment for all services rendered during her time at the home, which she could not afford), these women were shamed through the bodily act of birthing, ostensibly when no emotional intervention should be able to dissuade women from their rightful identity as mothers.

Anne Drapkin Lyerly (2006), a scholar of social medicine, argues that at the time of a delivery, a mother's sense of being connected rather than feeling abandoned, of being empowered, and of having dignity are "crucial" elements to having a positive birthing experience (103–4). Further, Lyerly contends that childbirth represents a "particularly critical locus" of pervasive cultural messages about women's polluted sexuality that comes to bear on her new identity as a mother, along with expectations of what proper womanhood and proper motherhood should be (111). These perspectives on how integral the birthing experience is to a mother's sense of herself *as a mother* provide a framework for listening to women's stories about delivery and the days after childbirth.

Discussions of what would happen during labor—the process of a body getting ready to give birth and the subsequent medical procedures that might be expected—were few and far between for young women who resided in maternity homes. Deborah remembers feeling somewhat prepared because of a book that she read about the process of giving birth, although she cannot remember where she obtained it. Pam recalls having no idea what to expect. Gayle explains that when childbirth was discussed, maternity home staff used vague and unspecific language that did little to actually prepare the women for labor. At some homes, women returned after delivering and thus had an opportunity to share their experience (or what part of it they remembered) with other residents. At other homes, going into labor meant leaving the home immediately and permanently. As part of a context of radial, radiating shame, childbirth marked the end of hiding, a vacuous experience at the end of a long, isolating time of waiting.

Obstetrics at mid-century was highly systematized by physicians at the expense of women giving birth. The nonconsensual use of anesthetics to administer "twilight sleep" and deliver a baby with forceps was a common obstetric practice from the 1930s to the 1970s (Clow 2003; Lyerly 2006, 107), and groggy, laboring women were commonly strapped down to delivery room tables (Wolf 2009, 11). In addition to these efforts at corporal management, physician's attitudes and actions toward unwed mothers reportedly could be inhumane. Barbara, a white woman who hid at home through her pregnancy, visited the same doctor as did her mother and married sister, who were also pregnant at the same time. Throughout her pregnancy, Barbara recalls: "I was convinced that this doctor hated me. Because from the first day he told me, 'I don't give anesthesia to girls like you.' Um, you know, he just looked at me with such disdain. So he would examine [my sister], and talk to her, and let her listen to the heartbeat. And when it came to me, you know, 'Let me feel you a little bit. Eh, everything is good.' Oh, it was horrible. But my mother had ten children and in her wisdom she did not agree with him on the anesthesia bit. So she sent a friend of hers, who was a registered nurse, and she was with me in delivery. And I remember her stroking my head right before I went out. And that was like the only kindness that I had during that process." This memory links the anticipation of labor without pain management with the degraded status of being pregnant and unmarried—a connection that resonated across numerous interviews.

Priscilla, a white woman who worked in a wage home, remembers that while she had prenatal care, "nothing prepared [her] for what was to happen" when she went into labor (quoted in Wilson-Buterbaugh 2017, 238). She recalls being "unceremoniously" left in front of the hospital by the wage-home employer's boyfriend. She recounts:

> I was stripped of my clothing and possessions, placed in a windowless,
> empty four bed ward being used as a storage room and told to stay put

and not come out. How long I was there I have no idea. There was no clock, no phone, no radio, no visitors other than medical personnel who would come and check my progress. No words were spoken other than to the effect of, "Well, aren't you proud of yourself now? Look where your slutty ways have landed you!" I was given no pain medication nor any comfort whatsoever. When my water broke, I didn't know what was happening. I went to the door and called for help. The nurse (a nun) came running down the hall yelling at me to "Get back in there! There are 'decent' women here having babies!" Then angrily, "Look at this mess you've made!" (Wilson-Buterbaugh 2017, 238)

Other mothers' treatment was similarly harsh but not communicated so directly. For example, Carol describes herself as "a frightened young [white] kid" when she prepared to give birth in 1961 at the age of 17. Carol's experience at the hospital during and after her delivery largely define her experience of shame, because of the difficulty she had during her delivery, which was breech. She remembers: "Of course they left me to labor alone. And I was screaming. And [finally] a nurse came in and was very rough: 'What's the matter with you?' And she looks under the sheet and sees a little foot and she is screaming, "Oh my God! We need a doctor in here!" Carol explains that even after the birth, she was singled out and treated harshly by the nurses at the hospital: "I never could understand why they treated me so badly in the hospital. When it came time to get—for the women to get their babies—because I was in a room of four—they brought the babies to the other three women but [the nurse] didn't bring my baby. And I had to ask for the baby. And she said, 'You want your baby?' It was a very down-the-nose treatment." It has only been within the last few years that Carol learned that many hospitals used codes like BUFA (Baby up for Adoption) to distinguish illegitimate or "unwanted" children and the women who were "giving" them away. This information suggests how morality encroached on the medicalized space of the hospital, revealing codes that distinguished patients and, likely, patient care. Such codes overwrote the patients and their experiences, indexing through shorthand the dispossessed status of shame-laden mother and child and the extractive measures taken to permanently sever an assumed shame-based mother-child relationship.

Even for women who received some level of attentive medical care during labor, the days after delivery were marked by isolation, as many women were not permitted to have contact with their child. "We were always encouraged to not hold the baby," remembers Gayle. "That was a big, big thing. I don't know who came up with that, but it was a big thing." Cynthia explains, "In the hospital, once I had him I didn't see him. They knocked me out. And I didn't get to see him. I knew it was a boy because I looked on my bracelet. I had been told before, at the home, that you are not going to see your baby. So I didn't ask." The maternity home staff convinced Cynthia, by telling her she could not see her child, that by getting pregnant outside of wedlock, she had surrendered her rights to be a mother.

The idea of surrendering one's child, sight unseen or seen only from afar, has its own rhetorical force, severing the mother–child bond in yet another radial aspect of shame. Barbara articulates the layers of separation, both physical and symbolic, between her and the child she had just delivered. "I wasn't allowed to see him. I got out of bed and I tried to find the nursery because I could hear crying. And I was met by a nurse who said, 'You are not allowed down there to see *the* baby.' It was always 'the' baby—there was never a pronoun like 'your' baby or 'your' pregnancy." Thus it was not merely a hallway separating Barbara and her child, but rather the imposed severance of identity, a motherhood seized. Cynthia and another unwed mother were able to "sneak down to the nursery" to see their infants. After identifying herself, Cynthia remembers that "the nurse just motioned to the back of the room. And that is where he was. I remember seeing him. I burned that image into my mind—with his blonde hair and his cute little nose. And I stood there as long as I could stand it before it was too painful. Then I had to walk away and go back upstairs. That was the only time I saw him."

These stories of unwed mothers' common experiences with delivery and forced postpartum separation reflect how such practices isolated mothers during and after labor and (with the use of drugs) both disconnected them *from* the physicality of the birth while also in many cases connecting them *to* physical and psychic pain. Mothers who shared with me their experiences of such pain considered it to be a method of punishment meted out by medical authorities. Such physical and emotional pain can also be an extension of radial rhetorics of shame insofar as pain that is individually felt can "rearrange bodies" and connect one body to a larger "world of other bodies" (Ahmed 2004, 28). Ahmed theorizes this sensational paradox, arguing that pain is "bound up with how we inhabit the world, how we live in relationship to the surfaces, bodies and objects that make up our dwelling places" (27). Pain as a differently felt aspect of shame distinguished the typical and expected pain associated with laboring bodies from that felt at the cusp of an unsanctioned, unrighteous birth. Pain replaced joy in the wake of childbirth's potentially universalizing and transcendental effects and functioned as a mechanism for rearranging a birthing person's relationship to motherhood despite and through the process of delivery and even the physical proof of her child. Such rearrangement has the potential to disrupt an embodied epistemology, or what Isis Marion Young (2005) refers to as a pregnant person's "bodily self-image of strength and solidity" (57) and the tendency for their subjective experience of pregnancy to involve experiencing themselves as "a source and participant in a creative process" or that one "*is* this process, this change" (54; emphasis in original).

Such activities and practices—strikingly similar across stories of white unwed mothers of this time—are an extension of what Luna Dolezal (2016) refers to as *body shame,* or an "intensely personal and individual experience" that "bridges our personal, individual, and embodied experience with the social and political world which contains us" (ix). I consider Dolezal's work to theorize body shame—which focuses intently on beauty norms, cosmetic surgery, and other manifestations of shame culture as it relates to gendered embodiment—alongside rhetorical embodiment theory. Specifically, mothers' experiences of being shamed and nearly erased while laboring and after delivery demand that those understanding radial shame "foreground" the "laboring body" (Chávez 2018, 244) as crucial to the affective rhetorical ecology that upheld righteous reproduction. The resulting substitution of one identity—mother, unmarried—for another—nonmother—happened through an almost unfathomable form of body shame exercised at the moment of birthing and through an arrest of meaning-making between mother and child.

Revirginalization as
Duplicitous Redemption

"It was November 28, 1966. It was the day of Truman Capote's Black and White Ball, which was at the Plaza—a few blocks away." Deborah struggles to recall details of the "numb" time she passed at a Manhattan maternity home given the phenobarbital-induced haze that clouded her awareness and ability to remember: "And so they got me into a cab. I think somebody came with me but I don't really remember. They induced me and I went into labor. And I remember it being dark. I remember being alone most of the time. And I remember there was a window. And I could see it getting dark. And the darker it got, the worse my labor got. And it was just, it was just awful. I don't remember being comforted. I don't remember, I just remember it being horrible, you know?" Deborah was "put out" just before she delivered and came to after her baby was born. The next day, a nurse brought her daughter. "So I was able to see her. She was gorgeous. She was 5 pounds, 11 ounces, I think. I got to hold her. I didn't get to feed her. And I remember it being very hazy."

And just like that, it was all over. "I don't know if my parents went and collected my stuff or whether they sent it—I don't know how that happened. But I remember I didn't go back to the girls. I just went from the hospital [to] home," Deborah explains. "But it was a pretty sad Christmas . . . I remember just being very numb, just very numb. And I then I went back to school in January."

Part of what defined this era as a time when unwed mothers knew, unequivocally, the shame of their transgression, was the need to pretend that the entire system of hiding never existed, that a birth never happened. As the final stage in rhetorically enacting a return to purity, a performance of revirginalization not only erased the physical reminders of illicit sex (namely a pregnant body or an infant), but metaphorically returned a mother to a presumed state of sexual innocence. In this case, such a state hews closely to the developmental stage of puberty, which can both connote purity and align with personal feelings of shame. Simone de Beauvoir theorizes puberty as a "*crisis*" for girls who, because of the social taboo of the menstruation as a marker of sexual maturation, enter it with a range of feelings including shame, disgust, fear, ambivalence, and/or pride (quoted in Young 2005, 100, emphasis in original). In addition to this fictive return to a renewed shame-prone state, unwed-mothers-as-now-revirginalized-women also coped with the loss of their children (along with possible postpartum depression) in silence.

Repeatedly the mothers I interviewed explained that once they returned home after giving birth, the subject of the pregnancy was strictly taboo. For example, Mary's father made plans for her to return home after her delivery because, in his words, "now" she was "*feeling* better." In most cases, there was simply no discussion of what happened, and this imposed silence carried great meaning. Cynthia explains: "I was totally lost when I came home because there was no counseling, there was no-one to talk to. If you lose a baby any other way—through a death or something—there are always people to surround you and support you. And I had nothing. My mother's only statement was, 'Hurry up and get a job. Get a job.' Because I had to pay for my stay at Catholic Charities . . . It was my crime and I was going to pay for it." The silence that surrounded Cynthia amplified rather than quieted her feelings of shame. Similarly, Barbara explains that she told her husband about her past when they got married, but otherwise, "I never told anyone. Because there was so much shame and so much guilt. That you just kind of bury it. And live your dysfunctional life. It is just a horror."

The imperative to never discuss such experiences communicated that even though these women had followed their family's or authority figures' advice perfectly, this method for repurification was only as good as their perpetual secret-keeping. Such requisite silence is a form of preemptive security against any additional disclosure for a family seeking and trying to maintain an outward presentation of normativity. Such preemptive security in these cases reveals the continued presence of shame because it is, according to Brian Massumi (2010), "predicated on a production of insecurity to which it itself contributes" (58). In other words, mothers' feelings of shame render her responsible for the emotional and cognitive burden of secret-keeping and the perpetual denial of her lived and embodied experiences. Because of the unrelenting demands of daughters' sexual purity as a demonstrable marker of the overall family status, the unwed mother's shame encumbers her with the responsibility of upholding the fictive and assumed (re)virginity narrative.

Enduring secrecy and silence, then, did not function as protection for these women, but as a haunting. Jackie explains that her family needed to keep her pregnancy a secret in order to protect her and them (as church members) from gossip. But Jackie explained that the secret-keeping actually fueled gossip, especially among the congregation. Receiving several anonymous phone calls upon returning home, Jackie listened with no recourse as a caller taunted and threatened; they knew Jackie's secret and why she held it. Also reflecting the pain of imposed silence, Barbara recalls returning from the hospital and being implored to celebrate her sister's new baby because, according to the family fiction, "this was a happy time." Emory University psychiatrist Irene Phrydas explained in 1964 that "the majority of the girls [who have a child out of wedlock] magically believe that all of their problems will be ended as soon as the baby is born" (9a). The statement hints at the inability of secrecy to truly erase a past, but Phrydas also attributes the magical thinking to naïve and chimerical girls. In contrast, the mothers' testimonies reveal that if the mothers did participate in such wishful thinking, they did so because, not in spite of, the silences that encased them. These young women lacked the knowledge that would enable them to predict the resounding, reverberating, and ongoing silences that would come in the wake of having their baby. In retrospect, most of the mothers speak of hiding and being forced to surrender a child in silence as a traumatic experience.[7] Mary simply repeated, throughout her interview, that the practice "destroys lives."

The flawed logic and practice of secret-keeping too often ruptures, as I have demonstrated throughout this chapter, suggesting that the promise of revirginalization, despite its superficial rhetorical affordances, could not offer a white mother or her personal network of loved ones any true redemption. Just because secrets are betrayed does not mean that they can be owned and wielded by those who have been silenced. Conversely, radial shaming's demand for a surreptitious "restoration" of purity has resulted in many mothers experiencing varying relationships to trauma and, further, a type of ontological failure—an ongoing sense of profound individual deficiency based on shame's situational effects in the short and long term. For those who experience trauma of the body and the psyche, secrets can also represent the "unsayable," that which can be too painful to remember and purposefully express. In her work with girls who have been sexually abused, psychotherapist Annie Rogers (2006) explores how trauma intervenes in language use, even when it is still known to the body. Rogers argues that the most unsettling aspect of trauma is not necessarily its connection to instances of abuse, but rather to "the way terror marks the body and then becomes invisible and inarticulate" (44). The internalized, destructive force of secret-keeping becomes evident in Deborah's explanation of coming back:

> They told us that we would go home and forget this . . . So, I thought I would forget about it, because that is what everybody told me. But I didn't. So then I thought there was something wrong with me, because everyone else seemed to forget about it. And so there was an inner sadness that you have. But it gets worse—at least for my generation it got worse for a couple of different reasons. If we went on to have other children, we realize what we have given up. You didn't realize—I had another child and realized what I had given up. And realized every time my other daughter reached a milestone I would wonder where [my first daughter] was and what she was doing. And then as society changed and it became more and more possible for women to keep children, you kind of wondered, "Well, why couldn't—why was I so meek? Why didn't I stand up? Why couldn't I—I should have been stronger. I should have been smarter. I should have known better." And so you get into this blaming game, you know? And part of the healing for me has been to realize that I'm strong now because of this.

Deborah told me that she has found healing, and that being able to share her story is evidence of this recuperation. "You pretend it [the birth] didn't happen," she explains, "And, you know, you can't do that." Along with noting Deborah's expression of such relief, it is crucial to avoid reading her experience as an expected resolution. Rather, relationships to healing or a lack of resolution vary and are unique to each woman's experience.

Radial rhetorics of shame, then, ultimately radiate back onto the unwed mother in ways that may not end, even though times and social norms change. Dianna Taylor's theory of humiliation as "internalization" helps to explain this radial return to a changed understanding of the self. Taylor (2018) draws on Michel Foucault's notion that humiliation ruptures ties with others, results in a break in one's relationship with oneself, promotes obedience, and diminishes the likelihood of emancipatory attitudes or actions. Her theory of internalization refers to "exposure and display before oneself, of an externally generated perception of oneself as radically individuated" and simultaneously not eligible for freedoms that would allow one to "become other than what one currently is" (440). This self-directed return of acute shame, then, facilitated pregnant women "adjusting" to their fate as erased mothers who would bear to-be-forgotten children. Some mothers' sense of dissonance when orienting to what can be read as mere complicity in child separation suggests the profundity of this shame at work. Mothers' feelings of ontological failure based on shame discouraged them from speaking out for themselves while pregnant; deterred them from feeling solidarity or seeking a collective, resistant, counterpublic voice; and arrested their ability to self-identify as mothers despite having physically given birth.

The "choice" to secret a pregnancy and continue to keep the secret for years thereafter is a complex one because of the women's extreme sense of disempowerment as allegedly illicit mothers. Those who I interviewed helped me to understand that in many cases, identifying oneself as a once-unwed mother is not simply speaking a long-unspoken truth but instead is an existential reckoning with one's supposed identity as a "bad" mother. The collateral damage has had a profound effect on many of the women with whom I have spoken. For Mary Ann, the messages of shame related to being an unwed mother "confirmed that I was a worthless person, an odd person. I always felt like I was odd. I still feel odd. Looked fat. Yes, [my unwed pregnancy] made it much worse. I felt like I was an outsider to the life that I lived before. But I was no longer entitled to be the person I thought I was going to be."

Hearing shame rhetorics as an indictment of the self is something that Audrey also experienced. Upon returning to her parents' home after giving birth and relinquishing her child for adoption, Audrey described herself as "a *persona non grata*. When I went home, I was not allowed to eat at the dinner table. I had to eat up in my room or in the basement. My brothers and sisters were not allowed to talk to me. You know, it was total isolation. Not—I mean—it was bad enough to be shunned at school. And ordinarily you go home because that's where you live and you have reasonable expectations that you are safe there and you are protected and it is a good place for you to be. That's not how my home was—at all."

As these memories suggest, shame contributed to an affective rhetorical ecology in which these women were unlikely to renegotiate the boundaries of propriety and reconfigure themselves as mothers in an alternate form. The power of these shaming rhetorics to shape one's sense of self was most apparent to me when I spoke with Elizabeth, a white woman from Euclid, Ohio who hid her pregnancy in 1961. During her interview, Elizabeth repeatedly assured me that she was "not sorry" for the pregnancy and adoption because she had "made a mistake and . . . paid for it." Elizabeth refuses to remain conscripted by shame because, according to her logic, she gave penance for an unrighteous act. She undercut her own affirmation by adding, at the end of the interview, "I hope you—I hope you don't think I'm a terrible person."

Rhetoricians have observed emotion's relationship to communicative ecologies and, more specifically, its ability to circulate and function as what Emily Winderman (2014) refers to as a "collectivizing" rhetorical force in her study of anger (386). Erin Rand (2014) also theorizes the rhetorical function of emotion as she compellingly writes about shame's "tremendous affective potential"

(138). Rand argues in her analysis of the AIDS activism group ACT UP that "the more powerfully felt the emotion and the more tenacious its roots in the constitution of particular identities and subjects, the greater its promise as a resource for agency" (138). Although this assertion aligns with Rand's project, it fails to represent the experiences of women featured here. What makes shame "sticky," then, when it threatens to shame people in proximity to unwed mothers but not "sticky" among unwed mothers who shared the experience of being physically ostracized, emotionally spurned, and subject to residual shaming over time?

Radial rhetorical shaming—a rhetorical mechanism that breaks women's sense of their identity (moral and social), agency, and rhetorical capacities—provides one answer. Radial rhetorics of shame are the reason that Mary Ann shared with me her feelings of rhetorical incapacity when she saw her son in foster care some time after giving birth—a situation that she realizes now was atypical for unwed mothers like her. Mary Ann concludes that she "still blew it" by not advocating for her own desires or needs as the mother of her "illegitimate" child. She recounts being "so afraid. I was so afraid that I was crazy, that I would be crazy forever. That I would never be able to take care of a child, or myself, or anything else. So I just went, I went passively along with anything anyone ever told me to do or not do." Similarly, Pam, who became pregnant at age 14 and who surrendered that child, admits struggling for years with the fear that her later children would also be taken from her. As she explains, "It was trapped in my brain . . . I was not allowed to be a mother" (Fessler 2007, 172).

The state of permanent arrest in recognizing the self as a mother—any type of mother—suggests that shame in service of righteous reproduction has "secure[d] the willing participation" of once-unwed mothers and thus reinforced their marginalization in their youth and, in many cases, throughout their lives (Rand 2015, 163). The residual and pernicious effects of radial rhetorics of shame in its many expressions thus simultaneously bolster the category of unrighteous reproduction while "reinforcing the structures that enhance the validity of [in this case righteous] others" (163). Some of the mothers with whom I spoke are active in adoption reform, participate in support groups related to adoption, or are otherwise open to publicly sharing their stories; yet nearly every woman described a long period of silence in the years after the pregnancy in which she chose to speak minimally, if at all, about her experience of going away. The fact that in several cases, mothers chose to contact me (one "after a glass of wine"), set up an interview time, and then decided against sharing their stories (a perfectly reasonable decision, of course) suggests that, at least in some cases, some women are still actively negotiating how they want to engage with and/or share these memories. Indeed, over the years of conducting this research I have received and still do get an occasional, typically brief, email that discloses the sender's identity as a woman who was pregnant while unmarried, who went away, and who has heard about my research. I always interpret these clipped, guarded messages as heavy with memory and, likely, grief—and despite my effort to respond by opening a space for listening, I have become used to no further reply, as these mothers may have decided against reopening a painful past.

Why Must Radial Rhetorics of Shame Be Understood?

I conclude each of my interviews with the same question: Why is it important for others to know about your story? "It is very important that the truth get out. Because of all the—I can't tell you how many times [I've heard] 'Oh, she didn't want that kid. She just wanted to go out and party!' And that is so far from the truth" explains one mother. Another shares, "I always love when someone is interested in our story and wants to tell it because not a lot of people are. Sometimes adoptees will get very flippant with 'Why didn't you fight? Why didn't you do this? What didn't you do that?' So it is so nice to see someone your age who . . . can see how absurd this was. And it was." In the words of yet another mother, "I think that there probably are women out there who are so afraid that they are just hurting themselves. They are just keeping in that kind of frozen state."

Contextualizing the process of hiding and surrendering a child for adoption can be incredibly instructive to those who learn about it now and find such processes completely foreign. Exploring how going away was operationalized through radial rhetorics of shame is one way to demystify this complicated history and understand white unwed mothers' constrained positions. Exploring the effects of shame, Bonnie Mann (2018) implores scholars to understand the emotion not as mostly or exclusively episodic but as pervasive and "unbounded"—"a thick, relentless, engulfing" feeling that has no redemptive end (403). Understanding radial rhetorics of shame helps to disentangle the various moves that result in once-unwed mothers' conscription in a scapegoating mechanism that resulted in the loss of a child and a mother identity. My efforts to detail the various aspects of radiating shame as rhetorically constructed also help to illuminate how shame "saturates social space" in such a way that, as Mann argues, "the subject does not undergo shame in an entirely lucid state." Mann continues, "shame discloses without resulting in a corresponding cognitive understanding of what is disclosed" (410). So while for some mothers, sharing their stories may be a product of their recognition of shame's lingering effects, for others it likely introduces new and partially explored relationships with the self.

Revisiting these stories brings them forward for public recognition and remembering. White women experiencing the shame of coerced relinquishment of a child have some similarities to women like Jean Whitehorse, who hid a reproductive-related violence (her involuntary sterilization)—though the violence of forced relinquishment and sterilization are profoundly different. Across these cases, women were denied the fundamental right to have a child and faced scenarios that compromised their dignity, safety, and well-being; these are all concerns of reproductive justice. Gathering and studying stories of these unequal violences is necessary feminist historiographic work, for as Glenn (2004) reminds us, "women's silence or the silence of any traditionally disenfranchised group often goes unremarked upon if noticed at all" (11). Writing her memoir about unwed motherhood, Moorman admits to feeling "an overwhelming sense of loneliness" because she believed "that no one could possibly understand what I had gone through, and that even if they did, they wouldn't care" (63). A similar theme rises in Whitehorse's story, which reflects her years of nondisclosure and reluctance to talk about what felt to her like an individual experience. As Adrienne Rich (1979) reminds, "Lying is done with words, and also with silence" (186).

An investigation of white reproductive righteousness as enacted through radial rhetorics of shame suggests how and why race- and class-based shaming practices bolster public notions of reproductive righteousness. Taylor (2018) argues that such profound experiences of shaming not only result in "radical individuation of victims" that compromise one's sense of selfhood and personal possibilities, but that such shaming also "shores up external relationships" including "those of the communities who close ranks around [the shamed]" (442). While this chapter sheds light on experiences of scapegoated white mothers, it also broadens understandings of righteous reproduction cultures and the white, upwardly mobile communities that radially benefitted from these multidirectional shaming practices. These same logics of familial normalcy, personal responsibility, and a sexual double standard indirectly informed population control programs and neo-eugenic programs that I discuss in more depth throughout this book.

Although shame emerged in largely consistent ways across mothers' stories, for Louise, the woman whose story opens this book, the operation of shame was slightly different. Shame was the reason she spent the last three months of her pregnancy in a Catholic Charities home for unwed mothers, why she relinquished her child for adoption, and why she was considered impure by peers who heard rumor of—or suspected—her pregnancy. The associations between righteousness, unwed pregnancy, and shame, I am confident, are the reason that she tells me she has held off seeking a reunion with her child, even though, she assures me, her later children—who do not know of her hidden pregnancy—would "be okay with it" because Louise and her husband raised them to be "open-minded" people. Unlike the experience of so many other mothers, however, Louise explains that her parents "were with me from the very beginning" and that her time at the home was not so much unpleasant as necessary. Louise also recalls a woman at the same home who arrived briefly before giving birth and who announced to the nuns upon arrival that she planned to take her child home with her. When I asked Louise, with surprise, if this woman was allowed to do so, she confirmed that she was, adding that the woman self-identified as also having been an "illegitimate child" who was raised by her unmarried mother. When the mother learned of her daughter's pregnancy, she put a plan in motion, instructing her daughter to bring the baby home where it could be raised with love.

Louise's memories prompt me to consider shame's presence at this slightly earlier postwar moment, to be mindful of its rhetorical malleability, and to critically imagine how purposeful rejections of shame-based scripts of gendered and raced sexual righteousness have the potential to enable personal agency, if not social change. In no way do I share these reflections to suggest that other mothers (or families) *should* have acted differently, as my conceptualization of radial shame has sought to evidence its ecological and enveloping—that is, exceedingly suasive—role at this historical moment. Nevertheless, Louise's recollections encourage heeding Nan Johnson's (2002) call: "the task of feminist histories of rhetoric implies not only identifying which women have been silenced or overlooked throughout the history of the tradition, but also pursuing just as dedicatedly information about why women are silenced and how programs of rhetorical silencing were deployed" (12). Just as important as listening to stories and imagining what is not or cannot be shared is theorizing how rhetorical practices of shaming are, in Mann's words, "unbounded" and "engulfing" across space and through time—how memories of the violences of going away are inviolable, permeable, and undisputedly enduring.

Two

New Permissiveness, Stigma, and Unwed Pregnancy in the Early 1970s

"Not so long ago, it used to be that when an unmarried girl became pregnant, her parents packed her off for a long visit to some faraway 'Aunt Martha.' Months later, her figure back to normal and her baby up for adoption, the unwed mother would return home, sadder but wiser." In March 1972, this recollection opened a *Newsweek* article, "Aunt Martha's Decline," which described changes in the openly secret culture of maternity homes. As detailed in chapter 1, these homes had long functioned as repositories for unwed mothers (often white) who hid an unrighteous pregnancy, typically surrendered their child as well as their identity as a mother, and participated in metaphorical and performed revirginalization. The article continues: "But times have changed. Today, the liberal attitudes that gave rise to the Pill and legal abortion have also made it possible for many unmarried women to bear children openly in their hometowns—and keep them. One casualty of this social revolution has been 'Aunt Martha,' the old-fashioned home for unwed mothers" (100). From *Newsweek*'s account, prudish Aunt Martha was now, by the early 1970s, a relic of the past. As noted more directly in one maternity home report, in the first few years of the new decade, "the need for a protected hideaway was gone" (McConnel and Dore 1983, 34). According to such sources, the intricate web of secrets and silences that had been constructed to avoid the radial shame a white unwed pregnant woman could bring to her loved ones were, within the span of only several years, unraveling.

What could account for such a change in white women's need for elaborate practices of hiding and surrender? A 1971 report prepared for the Birmingham, Alabama Salvation Army Home and Hospital for unwed mothers suggests that such institutions were posing this very question. According to the report, "the Army" continued to provide needed services, but there was an explanation for why only 70 percent of the Birmingham home's beds were full in 1971, as compared to the above-capacity enrollments the year before: "availability of

contraceptive information and materials," the "increased availability and acceptance of abortion," and the "changing community attitudes toward the unmarried mother and single-parent families" were to blame. "It is probably the
latter consideration [changing attitudes] that most seriously affects the intake
at maternity homes," the report continues. Anticipating misinterpretation of
data, given long-standing racialized and righteous reproductive logics, the report emphasizes that these attitudes did indeed apply to white unwed mothers
and not just Black unwed mothers. The caveat preemptively corrected what it
framed as an understandable point of confusion based on Black mothers' "statistical influence" on overall rates of unwed pregnancy ("Salvation Army" 1971).

These accounts reflect a concern that notions of sex as only sanctioned
within the confines of marriage were giving way to a new permissiveness of
the 1970s. The angst related to this supposed permissiveness suggests a concern
over sexual mores changing among white women—and specific fears about a
racialized spread of desire and a diminishing innocence of young white women.
New permissiveness—a spirit of sexual freedom and liberation connoting various forms of laxity in relation to sexual and bodily propriety, especially during
the late 1960s and early 1970s—handily explained why the era of hiding and
surrender began to erode. This justification for change did not quell, but rather
redirected, anxieties based on fears of US society's loosening allegiance to
norms of white supremacy, patriarchy, and class-status. (I discuss the other two
explanations—oral contraception and access to abortion—in chapter 3.) Spurred
by social movements of the late 1960s, ideas and practices of sexual freedom
gained traction and threatened to spread to (white, middle- and upper-class)
women across the nation who, some feared, might more openly consent to sex
outside of marriage.

I revisit the affective rhetorical ecology of this recent historical moment of
alleged new permissiveness with several key questions in mind. If young, white,
middle-class, unwed, and pregnant women were no longer necessarily beacons
of shame that threatened to radiate onto their families, if the cultural mandate
that they go into hiding to deny their motherhood and their child was not
being upheld with rigor, then how were these still-not-fully righteous unwed
mothers to be publicly present? How were they to be visible and understood?
And how were other women—poor and/or non-white women—perceived, and
later remembered or forgotten—in relation to this perceived cultural change?
In this chapter I demonstrate how a narrative of sexual permissiveness as moral
decline reshapes figurations of reproductive righteousness and serves as a mol-
lifying public account of social change. This explanation, when considered in
light of this recent historical context and together with close analysis of key
texts that index reproductive change, suggests a recentering of the righteous
desires of a majoritarian white and class-conscious nation that happens, in

part, at the expense of people (such as non-white women who were coercively sterilized) whose reproductive capacities threatened that worldview. More broadly, key stakeholders grappled with the shifting boundaries of righteous reproduction, as suggested by the emergence of a focus on "school-age teenage pregnancies" among social service and governmental agencies. Age served as a burgeoning and available factor for negotiating who in a modified context was un/righteous (and why) and how publics should subsequently respond. Relatedly, school (here meaning sites of public secondary education) became a critical backdrop for working out modified ways of configuring and responding to unwed pregnancy. These revised approaches to inscribing righteousness set the stage for wider *public* practices of punishment and protection that can and should be examined across racial, ethnic, and class lines.

An early 1970s public fixation on school-age mothers contributes to this study of gendered shame especially by illuminating shame's endurance and reconfiguration in more stigmatizing ways. Preoccupation with school-age women as reproducing bodies warranting management—more than just an indicator of practical considerations by, for instance, school administrators—is a reflection of a constructed scene of shame. As private shaming practices gave way to more public engagements with the "problem" of unwed pregnancy, a more scenic uptake contributed to how shame was rhetorically reconfigured and how it furtively lingered. In this altered context, shame links to a contagion-threat of the (raced and classed) innocence of white youth being endangered through proximity to unrighteous reproducing girls—an emerging class of stigmatized bodies. Judicial and legal efforts to officially manage and regulate unwed pregnant bodies within educational spaces suggest the pervasiveness of shame related to unwed pregnancy and its mutation into stigmatizing rhetorics that responded to morally contagious bodies.

It is true that even in the first years of the new decade, the mandate for going away was beginning to recede and the "problem" of unwed pregnancy became one of more open concern. More important than interrogating why the architecture of silence surrounding unwed pregnancy began to splinter, publicly, in this way is investigating how discourses surrounding these decisions constructed unwed pregnancy (or anticipatory fears of it) so as to discourage tolerance, later offer conditional tolerance, and—significantly—eventually frame legal protections for unwed student mothers-to-be. Such figurations rely on medicalized orientations that fail to explicitly confront the stigmatizing practices that necessitated legislation in the first place. They also provide emerging forms of support for long-standing racialized notions of protected childhood status being a priority for and a right of white children who connote an essential innocence while such childhood purity is denied to (for instance) Black children. Further, early case law from this period illustrates residual, well-articulated intolerance of unwed pregnant bodies, while later legislation written in the spirit of tolerance and inclusion relied on discursive constructions of unwed pregnancy-as-disability that do not decouple the unwed pregnant student (the source of rights claims) from her pregnant body (the source of ongoing stigma and shame) or to consider her as a rights-bearing student mother-to-be. These rights, however, were irrelevant to those women who were involuntarily sterilized, whose human right to have a child was already forever extinguished.

Centering stigma in this analysis of rhetoric, affect, and public emotion, I "follow through" on what shame does "at different levels," considering how various affects make us "feel, write, think, and act in different ways" (Probyn 2010, 74). I focus on stigma as a given/received feeling based on an ostensibly bad or abnormal body—one that is perceived to be attributable "proof" of a stereotype (Link and Phelan 2010, 366). Stigmatization as a process, then, helps to account for decisions being made about young, unmarried, pregnant, and reproducing women who were, at this point, more publicly present. Theorized by Erving Goffman (1963), *stigma* is a social practice applied to groups of people who are designated as different and inferior, and my analysis focuses on this difference resulting from some marked or visible status. As a rhetorical exercise of power, stigma articulates to classes of people who are designated as non-normative because of some shared quality (4). Stigmatization, like processes of shaming more generally, are intersubjective; that is, they are a matter of both those who act upon their own privilege to "mark, assign, stereotype, and frame issues, people, and situations in particular ways" as well as those who are the recipients of such accusations, neglect, silencing, or other forms of discursive, social, or physical violence (de Souza 2019, 18–19). To stigmatize is to shame in ways that have structural implications for groups of people (Link and Phelan 2010, 379) that emerge from the visibility of bodies as well as from the perception that these bodies can contaminate by proximity. These assumptions serve as the basis for containment and bodily management.

Drawing from these foundational ideas, I focus on how differential practices related to young reproducing women as well as public deliberation and legislation about pregnant, school-age students encourage attention to shame's endurance around notions of youth, space/proximity, fears of contagion, and strategies of containment. References to school-age pregnant students call attention to an emphasis on youth as a vexed identity, given shame-oriented connections between whiteness (as a racial category) and women's sexual purity that were disrupted by girls' pregnancy as proof of sexual encounter. Relatedly, references to school-age pregnant students call attention to the space of the school as a contested site of publicly unrighteous pregnant bodies. Such students are, at this historical moment, a stigmatized group of bodies because of the "mark" of their sexual activity. Tolerance of them is threatening to other youth in their proximity. By theorizing this shift in public rhetorical deployment of shame with a focus on what I deem an age-space-contagion nexus, I interrogate how this emotion "reworks how we understand the body and its relation to other bodies" and "the social" (Probyn 2010, 74). In relation to legislation that would, in theory, apply to all unwed, pregnant, school-age girls, stigma describes the way shame as emotion is operationalized to justify separationist practices that were thought to prevent unrighteous contamination.

In this chapter, I construct a context for understanding differential ways of managing women's fertility during this moment by applying a reproductive-justice and feminist-rhetorical inspired method of interlinking disparate women's stories. With this perspective-through-amalgam in place, I turn to case law and legislation that set the terms for young women's rights as student-age mothers-to-be. As rhetorical artifacts, such texts provide much-needed nuance for understanding how, slowly and unevenly, the architecture of silence related to unwed pregnancy began to break apart and become a public issue. These documents' rhetorical reliance on notions of the stigmatized body and its threat of proximal harm reflects the persistence of shame in light of the age-space-contagion nexus that framed deliberation as well as the discursive constraints on publicly discussing unwed pregnancy in a way that upheld young women's dignity and human rights as school-age reproducing people. In sum, I explain the ultimate failure to practice and legislate acceptance of various unwed pregnant mothers-to-be (or potential unwed pregnant mothers-to-be) on the simple and shame-irrelevant basis of their interconnected rights to have a child, to parent that child with dignity, and to continue their education. Across experiences I investigate in this chapter, I consider the impressibility of young people (i.e., the ability to be impressed upon through the threat of contagion and proximity), especially at the sight and in the presence of women's bodies that would have "displayed" sexual unrighteousness. Such impressibility warranted curtailing the rights of reproducing girls to ostensibly preserve the racially understood innocence of other primarily white, school-age children.

Bodies Tolerated or Tamed?
Four Takes on Unwed Pregnancy

What was it like to be unwed and pregnant—or potentially pregnant—in the early 1970s? Finding a generally singular answer to this question is impossible given the evidence of distinct attitudes and practices influenced by a woman's race, geographic location, socioeconomic status, and other factors. Laying alongside one another four stories related to unwed pregnancy demonstrates the uneven uptake (or total rejection) of the new permissiveness and provides a rich context for considering the varied stakes of sexuality, youth, and potential motherhood in a time of promise and lingering shame. Greater public attention to "school-age pregnancies" at this time prompts attention to wider gendered and racialized constructions and assumptions of youth and innocence—whether upholding long-held values or actively renegotiating them. For instance, the legal threshold for adulthood was lowered from 21 to 18 in many states over a five-year period starting in 1969 because of adolencents' "increased maturity" (Paul, Pilpel, and Wechsler 1974, 142). Although school-age, pregnant girls were likely younger than 18 and thus not directly affected by this decision, the shift in perception about when and by what measure a teen becomes an adult demonstrates that the question of how to interpret maturity was in flux. Simultaneously, racist foreclosures of Black childhood and innocence rendered an out-of-time adultification of some children that undergirds violence to poor and/or non-white women as I describe below.

Four "takes" on unwed pregnancy at the dawn of the new decade enable a reproductive justice-based approach to listening across varied experiences and for linking them to one another and to structural sites of power. Doing so enables a more holistically—if surely incomplete—approach to grappling with their significance. I specifically consider which women were denied the right to have a child (and why) and which women were enabled to have a child (and how that right was managed). The resulting tapestry of recent histories illuminates how righteous reproduction was being challenged, rewritten, and reified at a time when the shame related to unwed pregnancy was ostensibly dissipating.

In April 1971, high school student Judy Fay was featured on the cover of *Life* magazine as she stood before her class, delivering a report. Fay's classmates and her male teacher give her their attention. The focal point of the image is Fay's distended midsection, upon which she rests her notebook. The essay opens:

> In a public high school classroom, a 16-year-old student, eight months pregnant and unmarried, presents a book report. Her classmates and teacher are unruffled, for the quiet scene is an everyday event at Citrus High in Azusa, California—and elsewhere around the country where educators are taking a radical new approach to an old and painful problem. Until a few years ago, the nation's public schools dealt with teen-age pregnancies by expelling the girls or by putting pressure on them to leave. Many humiliated families arranged secret and illegal abortions for their daughters. Others sent them away to "visit relatives" or, if they could afford it, hid them in private nursing homes. (Woodbury 1971, 35)

The article continues by exploring Citrus High's program to address the "special educational, medical and psychological needs of teen-age mothers" (35). Citrus High sets itself apart from many public high schools in 1971, because it allowed unwed pregnant girls to remain in school during their pregnancy and also considered these mothers-to-be worthy of an education attuned to their unique needs. This cover story suggests to readers how life could and should be for young, unwed, pregnant women by 1971. Instead of averting one's eyes from Fay's pregnant body, the nation was encouraged to see her as a young woman with promise, with needs, and with the support of her school.

Examining the same story, Jenna Vinson (2018) argues that the picture of Fay centers her body and thus "deflects attention" from larger gendered and institutional practices that pregnant students would have faced (49). Readers see the problem of school-age pregnancy as "fitting *them* [pregnant students] into the school context" while suggesting situational "harmony" (49–50). Vinson explains how Fay's body offers rhetorical encouragement to make a particular kind of sense of this new and unfamiliar sight. She usefully critiques the piece's choice to not address systems of oppression that left many other young women (especially those who were poor and/or non-white) with meager support. The article nevertheless portrays an aspirational moment in which pregnant (white) women of school age were also invoked as mothers-to-be who could be entrusted to share educational space with their peers.

Fay's experience seems distinct from that of Audrey, a white woman (mentioned in chapter 1) who was concluding her senior year of high school in Akron, Ohio in that same year. Audrey bided her time until graduation, dealing with the "whispers and looks" of other girls who knew her ruptured secret: that she had spent the summer before her senior year at the Akron Florence Crittenton Home for unwed mothers. I interviewed Audrey to find out what "going away" was like for her at a time when a story about Fay suggested that the shame of unwed pregnancy was being eroded by increasing tolerance. Given an expanding permissiveness, why was Audrey bound by radiating shame? Audrey became pregnant at 15, after having sex for the first time with her boyfriend. Her father was convinced that her unwed pregnancy would shame the family, whose demonstration of respectability depended on her, the hard-working, obedient, middle child of seven. Despite Audrey's older sister, also an unwed mother, being permitted to remain at home and keep her baby, their father was incensed about Audrey's situation. He physically assaulted her mother for "letting" Audrey—the "golden child"—shame the family and decided that Audrey would be "sent away."

Audrey would be able to hide at the maternity home over summer recess from school, ostensibly aiding the family in keeping her pregnancy a secret. She explained:

> I went there in—right after school let out, which was in June. And I didn't really look pregnant. . . . I was six months pregnant and no one could

really tell. I went to the home, and [long pause] it was just so [pause] it was unlike anything I ever imagined. I mean, we were treated [pause] well, I would say, we were fed very well and we went to our doctor's appointments regularly. We had our vitamins that we took—however . . . you could not leave. Everything was locked. You could not walk out any door at any time on your own. And if you found a way—like during the day, if we happened to kind of sneak out the side door that the delivery person would use to bring in groceries and things, we might be able to sit on the stoop for a little while, but that was all the fresh air that we ever got. We were not allowed outside. And there was a big iron fence all around the whole home [and] an 8-feet tall iron gate. You could not get through it.

Unlike Fay, who was welcomed into her Californian high school classroom as an unmarried, pregnant student, Audrey literally remained within one of "Aunt Martha's" houses, secrecy and shame still shrouding her unwed pregnancy.

Although Audrey's sense of confinement stems mostly from her experience inside the home, a particular memory relates how her pregnant, white unwed body (and her residency at the home) was seen by others: "One day, it was really nice and sunny and we were begging our house mother to let us go [across the street] to Burger King and let us get some hamburgers for lunch instead of having lunch inside. And she said okay. So there were about six of us who went. We got our meals and we sat down at a table to eat. And the manager came over and he said, 'You, you aren't allowed to eat here. You're going to have to leave.' He said, 'We don't want your kind here.' He said, 'You're going to have to go back across the street.'" Audrey and the other residents were not just customers; they were, first and foremost, a group of unwed mothers, displaying their bodies in public and making visible their shameful situation. For that manager, concerned with maintaining a space pleasing to other customers, "across the street" marked a significant distance—a needed barrier between stigmatized, unwed mothers and those who remained outside the Crittenton fence. Thus, the street distinguished "there" from "here" but also reinforced the notion that that "there" is an "inside" for "those types of girls," whereas "here" remains an "outside" for "the rest of us." As Roxanne Mountford (2003) suggests, such material divisions are rhetorically significant and interdependent, for "outside and inside are forms of negation, writ in primitive spatial dimensions, long associated with social inclusion and exclusion" (23). Audrey's experience challenges the idea that a culture of permissiveness was sweeping the nation, erasing the shame of unwed pregnancy; her story suggests the extent to which even small changes to shame codes could elicit proclamations of shame's erosion, even when it remains a viable rhetorical, affective resource.

Audrey recalls the humiliation that she and the other mothers endured as they left the restaurant. "We were walking through the parking lot and of course there is the drive-through and there are people who are actually eating in their cars and stuff and they just called us all kinds of names. Threw stuff at us. It was awful. It was really awful. And it's like that 50 feet from the parking lot to the gate at the home—that seemed like it took forever, walking. It—it was awful." Unlike California high school student Fay, Audrey was not given the right to be a mother or the freedom to venture outside the confines of the maternity home. Her body needed to be quarantined; the proof of her indiscretion, if seen in public, communicated tolerance of her unrighteousness.

Life's depiction of a "quiet scene" in Southern California and Audrey's experience of stigmatizing shame can be read alongside yet another salient experience in school-age women's reproduction in the early 1970s. Although a long-held practice inflicted upon poor, disabled, and/or non-white women, coercive or involuntary sterilization began to draw wide public attention by 1973.[1] That year, national news coverage broke of government-funded, nonconsensual sterilization programs. Attention to this practice galvanized around Minnie Lee Relf (age 14) and Mary Alice Relf (age 12), Black sisters from Montgomery, Alabama who were given tubal ligations without their knowledge or informed consent or that of their parents. The Relf story made headlines because both girls were young, because one of the girls had a (confirmed) developmental disability, and because the girls' mother, who did not know how to read, placed an "X" in lieu of her name on a form that she thought was consenting to birth control shots. Lonnie Relf, the girls' father, was out of town and not contacted by the agency when its staff obtained this "permission." The Montgomery Community Action Agency, responsible for the subsequent sterilization procedure, was a federally funded entity that provided "family planning" for recipients of Medicaid—including minors—who requested such services. The director of the agency's family planning efforts reported that the Relf "'family was well aware' of the sterilizations and 'was very pleased to have [the procedure done] at that time'" ("82 Sterilized" 1973). Lonnie Relf disagreed, and with the support of the Southern Poverty Law Center, he filed a lawsuit seeking $1 million in damages on behalf of his daughters (Thompson 1973). Additionally, the Relfs's experience prompted a class-action suit filed on behalf of more than 125,000 other "poor, minor, or disabled persons" who were involuntarily sterilized through federally funded programs (Charmallas 2009, 1126).

The story of the Relf sisters grabbed the attention of those unaware of or heretofore largely unconcerned with such racist and eugenic practices. The sisters' experience prompted public discussions about the function of sterilization among those deemed "unfit" to parent as well as about the role of social workers who were considered to be intermediaries between those receiving federal benefits and a government potentially desiring female recipients' sterility. The Montgomery Community Action Agency, facing national media scrutiny, admitted to also having sterilized "at least" nine other women, eight of whom were Black (Watkins 1973). As Dorothy Roberts (2017) shares in *Killing the Black Body,* the Relf lawsuit exposed the "shocking magnitude of sterilization abuse in the South" and led to estimates of 100,000–150,000 "poor women like the Relf teenagers" being sterilized each year by programs receiving federal aid (93).

Significantly, the agency responsible for the Relf sisters' sterilization based these decisions not on actual conditions but rather on the anticipation that these girls would likely bear children out of marriage and, subsequently, rely on state support. According to historian Rebecca Kluchin (2009), agency records reveal that by the early 1970s, "some family planning clinics had begun to sterilize 'unfit' girls who, they predicted, would become unwed mothers" (101). Thus, one of the "most striking features of sterilization demographics" during the 1970s was the extremely young age of those being sterilized, many of whom had not yet reached puberty (Ordover 2003, 168). The Relf sisters' experience represented only one portion of a much wider effort to enact sterilization abuses on not-fully-autonomous women, whose reproduction was being managed by authorities who sometimes acted with penal intent and unmitigated presumption. This dismal site of reproductive regulation is tied up in the management of young bodies because it was anticipated that they would reject dependence on a husband in favor of state-sponsored dependence.

A fourth perspective offers less clarity but nevertheless provides a necessary window into reproductive actions of this same time period. Specifically, it relates to a concerted, government-sponsored mass sterilization program in the United States that operated at the state level and was directed at poor women including Indigenous women, women of Mexican descent (many living on the West Coast) and women of Puerto Rican descent (many living on the East Coast). In relation to Indigenous people, majoritarian fears of overpopulation among the poor was intimately linked to Indian Health Service (IHS)-initiated sterilizations in 1970. Begun just five years after first offering family planning services to Indigenous communities (Lawrence 2000, 402), this program of compulsory sterilization was an effort to control "undesirable" populations through a neo-eugenic approach. An unknown number of women were involuntarily or coercively sterilized across various reservations and communities, as government reporting did not account for consent procedures. Despite a 1974 moratorium on sterilization of people under the age of 21 and/or who were deemed mentally incompetent by a physician, "Indian health professionals" increasingly took up an activist role, pressuring the US government to investigate ongoing sterilization activity (Theobald 2019, 156–58). These activists could not know the ultimate intentions for negligence on the part of authorities or what percentage of sterilizations were truly involuntary, but they agreed that such unethical practices needed to cease (163–64). Collectively, their efforts suggest how sterilization was a layered and emotionally saturated experience of fertility being managed (consensually or coercively) that had profound individual and communal implications (160).

Although it is inadequate to have one story stand in for the varied experiences of the many Indigenous, Chicana, and Latinx women who suffered coercive sterilization, leveraging the still-obscure story of several Northern Cheyenne women illuminates this site of loss, knowability, and unknowability. Former chief tribal judge of the Northern Cheyenne, Marie Sanchez, investigated how this issue might have affected her reservation, located in Montana. Like other activists, Sanchez used knowledge of allegations and emerging lawsuits to direct her investigation. She learned that among the Northern Cheyenne people, thirty women were sterilized between 1973 and 1976 (Torpy 2000, 9). Included in this number were two young women under the age of 15 who were sterilized after being told that they were receiving an appendectomy (9). The details of these two women's experiences remain blurry.

Other sterilization stories of Indigenous women have been more fully recuperated. For instance, Lorna Tucker's 2018 documentary, *Amá,* mentioned briefly in chapter 1, centers and recovers the story of Jean Whitehorse, a Navajo woman who has just recently shared her first-hand experience of being involuntarily sterilized in 1970 after her forced relocation to Oakland, California as part of a colonial effort to divest Native peoples of traditions, cultures, languages, familial networks, spirituality, and relationship to land. But the stories of young women recorded through Sanchez's investigative and legal efforts enable more focused attention on the systematic silences and erasures of these sites of reproductive violence in the name of population control—a euphemism for intentional racist and genocidal activity.

My reading about these young and unnamed Northern Cheyenne women and the inconsistency of the little extant evidence about a procedure that they endured that rendered them unable to bear children, prompts me to use "critical imagination" to consider how these fragmented stories can help to illuminate the yet-unknown, the potentially forever-to-be-unknown. Jacqueline Jones Royster and Gesa E. Kirsch's (2012) concept of "critical imagination" is a method for moving beyond evidence, or what can be known, to subsequently "think between, above, around, and beyond this evidence to speculate methodically about probabilities, that is, what might likely be true based on what we have in hand" (71). How did these young women learn about what happened to them? How did they grapple with the consequences of this violence? How did it shape their sense of self and their relationship with their families, their communities? Critical imagination enables posing these questions in light of Jane Lawrence's contention that compulsory sterilization was not just a matter of motherhood rendered unavailable to Indigenous women (although that site of erasure is profound in its own right, to be sure). Such practices "harmed the relationships between Native Americans and the government and between tribal communities, husbands and wives, and mothers and their children" (Lawrence 2000, 414).

For instance, *Amá* briefly mentions an unexpected coming together of two US Indigenous tribes to resist the Dakota Access Pipeline. The documentary (Tucker 2018) explains that long-standing differences between these two tribes—Crow and Standing Rock Sioux—are not unrelated to the steep reduction in childbearing and children within nations that were violated through sterilization abuse. With fewer people, each tribe had less means of resistance to oppression and had greater struggle, which has led to intratribal division. Additionally, throughout the film the women being interviewed express that they did not know about other women's sterilization—even if those women were family members and/or friends. Whitehorse's recollection of her own experience suggests further unknowability: she notes that she long thought she was the only person to have been sterilized against her will and that she chose to remain silent for many years because of the spiritual ramification of her situation. Navajo understanding of wealth as having children opposes the notions of wealth as economic and material accumulation that allegedly undergirded the entire program of compulsory sterilization directed to women living in poverty. Whitehorse admits feeling ashamed of her situation and links other life struggles to her sense of loss because of the sterilization. Tucker's narration includes the assertion that "so many [Indigenous women] have taken their stories to their graves [that] we'll never know the full extent of the suffering and the number of women affected."

Long-time silence holders among Indigenous communities have similar experiences to other abused women, such as those from the Mexican immigrant community who came together to resist sterilization abuse in the 1975 class-action lawsuit *Madrigal v. Quilligan*. The suit, filed against the Los Angeles County USC Medical Center on the basis that the facility was coercively sterilizing Spanish-speaking mothers, led to a 1978 ruling that absolved the hospital of liability on the contention that there was a simple breakdown of communication between patients and doctors. Like *Amá*, the film *No Más Bebés* (Tajima-Peña 2015) centers the stories of women involved in the lawsuit. One, Consuelo Hermosillo, reflects on initially resisting involvement in the lawsuit because her sterilization was such a painful secret. She admits not sharing her decision to take part in the lawsuit with her husband and traveling by bus to the courthouse alone, "angry, ashamed and afraid" (Valdes 2016). These feelings persisted after the ruling, and Hermosillo did not connect with the other plain-tiffs. The parallels of the elective and imposed silences and of feelings of shame experienced by Hermosillo and Whitehorse are noteworthy and instructive. Although I resist drawing unfair or hasty parallels between these non-white women's experiences and those of Audrey and other white women I write about in chapter 1, a connectivity related to experiences of shame can help situate all of these women within a larger landscape of reproductive violations that variously include rhetorical, spatial, affective, and physical dimensions.

Taken together, these stories of unwed women—two white women who were actually pregnant and several non-white women whose humanity was reduced by recasting them as embodied economic threats because of the pos-sibility of their future pregnancies—illustrate a fundamental truth: that in the early 1970s, the shame, stigma, and judgment related to unwed pregnancy did not merely dissolve and give way to an era of new permissiveness. Although this claim is not especially surprising, it is important to clarify and consider. Women still hid, women were still coerced into relinquishing a child they birthed, women were punitively or proactively sterilized, and women—many women—still felt shame and experienced silence instead of freedom, tolerance, or basic human rights, albeit for a variety of abuses. This is an important con-textual reality that must be understood in order to reframe and better under-stand the history of reproductive-related and sexualized, body-oriented shame to which this book prompts readers to bear witness. The notion of expanding permissiveness provides an uncomplicated and erroneous story for how many women, including unwed mothers, were treated during a time of great social change.

This contrastive set of stories demonstrates how sexual shaming is part of the maintenance of girlhood innocence as a raced construction, more read-ily available to some white girls than to their non-white counterparts. At this moment, when permissive sexuality was feared by some people in the United States, girlhood was ostensibly open to refiguration. Here I push to consider how the range of experiences described above collectively point to girlhood as an identity that does and does not align to biological age. As a messy identity category, girlhood in these examples does not necessarily refer to a state of pre-menstruation. That is, the Relf sisters were involuntarily sterilized while they were girls because of the already-extant fear of their reproductive capabilities as almost-women. At the same time, Judy Fay is resituated within the space of the school with the effect of visually demonstrating her nonthreatening status as a student. This move in some ways renders Fay relatively more girl-like and innocent than the Relf sisters or unnamed Northern Cheyenne women.

Despite my use of the terms *woman* and *women* throughout this book, I find it critical to explore the rhetorical trappings of these recent historical framings (and activities) regarding girlhood for several reasons. First, not doing so performs a troubling conflation of Black girls and Black women that, according to Aria S. Halliday (2019), is a typical move in "cultural rhetoric" (8). This conflation is one Halliday mostly discusses in relation to how Black women speak to one another, but it upholds her point, relevant to this study, that both academic and popular discussions of Black people and their experiences infrequently center Black girls (8). Additionally, as Robin Bernstein (2011) argues about childhood, the identity category into which I would place girlhood as a gendered construct, there is a connection between innocence and the child that is not only historically locatable and constructed but also "raced white" (8). Bernstein's work traces how by the second half of the nineteenth century, white girlhood (and white childhood more generally) enjoyed a synecdochic relationship to innocence: "to invoke white childhood was to invoke innocence itself" (63). Black children, including Black girls, were, in contrast, increasingly understood as being unable to feel pain by this time. This "sharply bifurcated" vision of "American childhood" resulted in white girls being considered as deserving of protections while Black girls were configured as sources of labor who were "emptied" of innocence (63) and thus denied childhood and even humanity (68). This earlier configuration of childhood as racialized coheres around understandings of innocence, protection, and pain. This linkage is relevant to this early 1970s moment and to rumblings of a permissiveness that threatened to further intertwine childhood and adulthood, white-raced innocence and Black-raced lasciviousness. Thus, all of the young women's stories shared above are usefully contemplated alongside one another, as representations of girlhood and mandatory "adultification" (Halliday 2019, 7) at this critical moment.

The Relf sisters' inhumane and "casual" sterilization, once recognized and determined to be a "scandal worth reporting" by the media (Davis 1983, 215), garnered national attention that amplified concerns over compulsory sterilization programs, even while other non-white women's and girls' experiences of the same brutality were largely ignored. Angela Y. Davis writes that the Relf sisters' story is "horrifyingly simple" and linked to sterilization abuse in Alabama, North Carolina, and South Carolina (216–17). None of these girls should remain, in the words of Saidiya Hartman (2019), "surplus women of no significance, girls deemed unfit for history and destined to be minor figures" (xv). Yet, a nation shocked at the knowledge of sterilized children did not feel sufficiently moved toward action. While these atrocities happened, school-age women not suffering such grave abuses and who became pregnant were still a "problem" to be solved. As the nation hesitatingly experimented with the idea of (some) unwed, pregnant bodies "going public," it would also have to face the challenge of articulating defensible stances on the rights and freedoms afforded or denied these young, expectant women.

Stigma at School: Pathologizing Rhetorics
and the Path to Legal Rights

Turning to legal protections for school-age girls and the arguments that enabled them also means foregrounding spatial and visual politics related to unmarried, pregnant students being seen at school. In 1963, a federal "specialist" on "services to unmarried mothers" captures the shame-steeped context most pregnant students in junior or senior high would face:

> Some schools discharge a girl when her pregnancy becomes known and provide no means of continuing education through home instruction or any other plan. Limited educational opportunities may be due to lack of motivation by the unwed mother and her parents, economic privation, community pressures or attitudes, and stigma or punitive school policies that virtually prohibit return to school. Any girl who is absent from school for any length of time will find it difficult to return. She will have feelings about being behind in her class and will have lost out socially as well. It is not strange therefore that the girl who has additional problems which carry a stigma will not return to school "on her own." (Gallagher 1963, 403)

Four years later, that same specialist noted the continuation of such constraints and expansions in the tutoring and special "day-school" programs for "homebound" and "pregnant and unmarried girls" (Gallagher 1967, 3). At the same time, a larger professional conversation around who held responsibility for educating young people about sex was taking place, the primary obstacle to school-based sex education being the dual fears of "harsh public criticism" and "the sex impulse itself," which, according to "widespread belief" was uncontrollable and "will, at the slightest opportunity, express itself in irresponsible, exploitative, damaging behavior" (Kirkendall and Cox 1967, 137). The hint of sex and the threat of the marked, sexualized body was so feared that not even married teachers could continue their work if they were known to be pregnant. Students rumored to be pregnant could be expelled and bore the burden of proving otherwise (Fessler 2007, 72). The presumptive contagious effects of the defiled, pregnant, student-age body—a body that would inevitably betray observable "proof" of righteousness—and the uncontrollable impulses of barely containable bodies on the verge of sexual excess threatened to imperil the sanctity of the school, which a larger public depended on as a space for managing desire.

School-age pregnancy in the early 1970s must be contextualized within the longer shadow of school as a politicized space after the 1954 *Brown v. Board of Education of Topeka* ruling and the delayed, then tumultuous, experiences with school desegregation. Jill Locke (2016) argues that integration not only prompted a shift toward thinking of schools as political spaces but also that through it "children became citizens in their own right—agents of social and political change and partners with adults in the quest for school equality" (137). Locke further surveys African American perspectives on desegregation and some white people's resistance to it to amplify the contention that such opposition to integration was primarily based on a white supremacist fear of interracial sex (154). White southerners who opposed desegregation argued fervently that segregation was divine law that would be met with divine punishment if reversed and that integration was a communist plot to destroy the United States (Dailey 2020, 223, 230). Panic about the possibility of interracial intimacy reflected white fears of loosening social regulations on sexuality that had, since the time of US slavery, denied Black men access to white women while giving white men access to all women. Such racist social codes—those related to sex and support for white men's exclusive, sanctioned access to white women— fueled white supremacy, upheld the taboo of interracial sex and intimacy, and justified the extraordinary violence of lynching (219–20). Anti-integration images circulating in the late 1950s depicted these gendered and racialized fears in telling ways—for instance, in depictions of "little white girls forced at federal bayonet point into the arms of African American schoolmates" (236).

Such fear, though racist and irrational, justified a consciously developed logic of good shame. As Locke (2016) describes, "many white parents and clergy believed that a strong sense of shame—a restraint and brake that involved students imagining themselves being judged by others—needed to be cultivated in children with the goal of sexual regulation" (155). This point has also been forwarded by Candace Epps-Robertson (2018), whose analysis of Virginia Senator Harry F. Byrd's discourse demonstrates his central role as an architect of desegregation resistance in the name of states' rights and civic responsibility through the prevention of race-mixing (36). The "regulative work of shame" was most evident in the South. There, coordinated pro-segregationist efforts reflected a will to reaffirm shame's role in maintaining a particular social order even as its efficacy as a public emotion *able* to uphold supremacist beliefs was being threatened by increased equity and acceptance (Locke 2016, 155–56). The struggle over desegregation, which because of debates around "bussing" extended publicly well into the 1970s, suggests how young, frighteningly sexual bodies were managed in public schools, offering an informative context for debates over pregnant students' rights. In both cases, students' bodies were ostensibly managed through the practice of segregation, their desires were ostensibly managed through a white supremacist logic of righteous reproduction in service of racial purity, and their emotions were ostensibly managed in service of using sexual shame as a tool for preserving racial hierarchies.

A 1971 article in the *Journal of School Health* presents "the problem of pregnant school-age girls" as "one of concern to every school system in the country" (Howard 1971, 362). Expelling pregnant students is an injustice that runs counter to educational goals, the author contends, because girls who remain in school are statistically more likely to graduate and improve their grades in the process. Nevertheless, few schools enabled ongoing access to education, those that did typically provided a paltry two hours per week, and some prolonged re-enrollment after delivery or prohibited it altogether (361). Further "social handicapping" occurred when "welfare systems" more frequently supported girls who dropped out of school than those who continued their education (363).

Charting judicial and legislative decisions of the late 1960s and early 1970s demonstrates that the debate about whether school-age girls should be permitted to attend high school during or after their pregnancies remained a contentious one. Scholars have largely ignored the two primary pieces of case law that contributed to establishing unwed student-mothers' legal rights to attend school. Additionally, the piece of legislation that protects those rights for all—Title IX—has been historically investigated primarily for its relevance to women's sports. Examining these documents together illustrates that although unwed mothers were given the legal right to remain in school with Title IX in 1972, previous rulings made evident the acceptability of denying pregnant girls admission to high school or the normalcy of this practice. Further, the reluctance among courts of law to protect the educational rights of pregnant students foreshadows many school administrators' resistance to upholding Title IX. These early pieces of case law rhetorically depict pregnancy as a source of contamination, while the later legislation crafts a discourse of pregnancy-as-medical-disability. Such pathologizing language distinguishes school-age, pregnant bodies as not "normal" at the same time that these discourses outline girls' legal protection to remain within the normative space of the US public high school. Thus, while pregnant women were ultimately granted legal access to the high school classroom, the understanding of their participation in this space is framed by discursive pathology.

First as contagion and then as disability, pregnancy here is framed as primarily bodily difference that perpetuates stigmatization and thus obliquely discredits the (often unwed) student mother's humanity as the basis of her identity. Pregnant students expelled from school represent motherhood erased from the visually cohesive message of school as a place of bodily control and white (female) sexual purity. Such dismissals also represent motherhood disrupted because pregnant students were singly held responsible for "their" offense and prevented the ease—perhaps the possibility—of completing their secondary education, a limitation that surely compromised their self-sufficiency. Two legal decisions illuminate the perceived threat of unwed pregnancy, a threat to which Title IX indirectly responds but which it does not articulate.

Clydie Marie Perry: Unwed Mothers Are "Dismissed"

In January 1969, the United States District Court in Oxford, Mississippi heard the case of *Clydie Marie Perry et al., v. Grenada Municipal Separate School District et al.,* a ruling that reinforced the belief that unwed, pregnant girls posed a legitimate threat to high school environments. Perry, a 17-year-old junior described in one newspaper article as being "poor and black," sought an injunction on behalf of all school-aged, unwed mothers in Grenada County (Rowan 1969). Perry unsuccessfully petitioned her local school board to attend school as an unwed, pregnant student. Although Perry claimed that the practice of "exclusion of a mother of an illegitimate child" was enforced on a "racially discriminatory basis," the Court's first action was to overrule the motion for an injunction based on the fact that "excluding unwed mothers [from school] is enforced in a nondiscriminatory manner without regard to race, creed or color." In Oxford, all unwed, pregnant students were unwelcome at school.

This decision, however, provided an opportunity for the Court to explain why nonadmittance of pregnant students was justified. (The Court ultimately posited that a girl who had only one illegitimate child should eventually be considered for readmission so that she might "rehabilitate herself.") According to District Judge Orma R. Smith, "the Court can understand and appreciate the *effect* which the presence of an unwed pregnant girl may have on other students in a school." He adds that "the purpose for excluding such girls is *practical* and *apparent*" (emphasis added). Smith's assuredness that all young people have the right to an education conditional on their righteous behavior parallels his confidence that unwed, pregnant girls are, nevertheless, a "bad influence." The ruling required that school boards allow the unwed mother to present herself at a "fair hearing" before "school authorities" who would reassess her moral character, since she still threatened to "taint the education of other students" (*Perry v. Grenada Municipal Separate School District* 1969). Thus, Smith endorses school administrators as the arbiters of moral worth for one-time offenders and reifies the notion that exile from school while pregnant is reasonable.

Smith's ruling illustrates a rhetorical and legal instantiation of contamination logics that reflects the desire to protect the greater student body from being tainted by the unwed, school-age mother. Impressibility as theorized by Kyla Schuller (2018) is a sentimental biopower that has been "hiding in plain sight," a "capacity of a substance to receive impressions from external objects that thereby change its characteristics" (6–7). Impressibility is an affective and sensorial aspect of the conceptual notion of contagion and proximity harm. According to education policy scholar Wanda Pillow (2004), the theme of contamination "circulates the idea that the presence of a sexually active female student (as a pregnant student or a mother) will contaminate the student body leading to an epidemic of immoral and promiscuous behavior" (63). This rhetorical depiction of "bad" pregnancy as infectious renders the unwed, pregnant body a viral threat to the well-being of impressionable others. Thus, this body must be contained away from the school, a symbolic site of purity and normativity. When the "normal" and the "stigmatized" come into contact, a confrontation, or reckoning, must occur (Goffman 1963, 13).

School administrators' typical practice of expelling pregnant girls sidesteps this confrontation and reinforces a practice of gendering that holds women wholly culpable for putatively unrighteous behavior. The designation of stigmatized female bodies and the related shame of that stigma function as a process of gendering—the process of learning the social constructedness of gender around, in this instance, reproductive responsibility, suppression of desire, and the embodied consequences of sexual activity. Such separation of contaminated bodies from noncontaminated bodies and spaces also functions to designate both the "marked" or "diseased" and the "pure." Representations of contamination and containment perpetuate a central fiction: that a stable body and identity can resist such invasion. The fact that female and pregnant students were viewed as a singular threat to the expectations of righteous (i.e., nonsexual-if-female) student bodies evidences a gendered stigma; the obviousness and alleged practicality of Smith's ruling points to the reified and publicly shared logic of this decision.

Discourses of contamination like those in the ruling function as metaphors of irrationality for unspoken economies of stigma that project meaning onto both bodies and spaces. Here, "normal" (i.e., nonpregnant) high school students are *stigmaphobes,* or those who belong to a dominant culture of nonstigmatized people. Conformity among stigmaphobes "is ensured through fear of stigma" (Warner 1999, 43). As Michael Warner explains, the "stigmaphile space" is the space of abnormality; it allows one to find "commonality with those who suffer from stigma." In contrast, the realm of the stigmaphobe is a space where normalcy reigns and where all cues, visual and otherwise, uphold this paradigm of invisible, taken-for-granted normalness. Thus, by barring admission of unwed pregnant girls, school administrators punished those "wayward" students who were "in trouble" by sending them "away" to some other stigmaphilic space—thereby preserving the school as a stigmaphobic, or normal, place. As a public and disciplinary site, the school importantly establishes and adheres to the boundaries of normalcy as productive regulation. Locke (2016) argues that the positive cultivation of shame was seen as a good among white parents and clergy who hoped for sexual regulation because of the covert affective suasion of "students imagining themselves being judged by others" (155). Casting unwed girls out of school functioned as stigmatizing that employed shame as a positive, functional emotion articulated to education.

Although the *Perry* case offers a window into considering rhetorics of contagious bodily shame at work in an initial instance of case law, it is imperative to attend to its application to a school-age Black girl, given extant fears of school-based "race-mixing" in this post–*Brown v. Board* moment. Locke (2016) argues that segregation portended legitimized "interracial love and friendship" that would ostensibly mark "the death of shame, once and for all" (155–56). If supposedly already hypersexual and ostensibly shame-resistant Black girls could be allowed to be pregnant in the space of the school, then the fragile if enduring linkage between whiteness, femininity, and regulative sexual shame could be undone. Unmitigated dismissal of unwed mothers reflects how administrators employed defense by avoidance, minimizing potentially explosive rhetorical situations by simply denying pregnant bodies access to an education and thereby "protecting" the more important student body from a threat of shameful contamination during this era of "permissiveness."

Ordway v. Hargraves: *Inroads Toward*
Unwed Mothers' Educational Rights

Another legal battle over the rights of unwed pregnant students was unfolding in Massachusetts when, in 1971, a white, unwed, and pregnant senior honor student, Fay Ordway, was granted permission by a District Court to continue to attend North Middlesex Regional High School. Ordway's mother brought a civil action on behalf of her daughter after Fay was dismissed earlier that year. Fay had informed Principal Robert Hargraves of her pregnancy in late January, indicating that she was due in June. Claiming that he was bound to enforce school board policies, Hargraves decided that Fay could not attend classes, could only use school facilities such as the library after the daily dismissal of other students, but could participate in some other school and senior-class functions. Fay requested a hearing, and a school committee upheld the decision (*Ordway v. Hargraves* 1971). In his testimony in District Court, Hargraves admitted that Ordway's pregnancy had not, despite fears to the contrary, disrupted the Middlesex educational environment.

Ordway v. Hargraves resulted in the District Court ordering that Ordway be permitted to return to school, a greater acknowledgement of the educational rights of unwed pregnant students than had come from the *Perry* ruling. Nevertheless, the account of the proceedings makes apparent the extent to which Ordway's unwed, pregnant, female body was considered a violation of the fictive, normalized, asexual space of Middlesex High. The ruling notes: "It is clear from the hearing that no attempt is being made to stigmatize or punish plaintiff by the school principal or, for that matter, by the school committees. It is equally clear that were the plaintiff married, she would be allowed to remain in class during regular school hours despite her pregnancy." Ostensibly, Ordway's pregnancy was not the problem at hand; her unwed pregnancy, rather, was the incriminating factor. Because the ruling insists that Ordway is not being treated in any unusual way, it demonstrates the extent to which Fay, a high school honor student, had disappeared in the eyes of the school committee and the Court. She was eclipsed by her status as an unwed pregnant girl with a visibly pregnant body, and thus, she represented a potentially ungovernable symbol of sexual deviance.

The unmanageable, rhetorical power of Fay Ordway's unwed pregnant body seems to have been more of a concern to school officials than any actual problems that arose while Ordway was still in school. According to the ruling, Ordway testified that "she has not been subjected to any embarrassment by her classmates, nor has she been involved in any disruptive incidents of any kind." Additionally, Ordway testified that "she has not been aware of any resentment or any other change of attitude on the part of the other students in the school" (*Ordway v. Hargraves* 1971). Several witnesses offered that the exile of a pregnant student could be detrimental to her and her baby's health. Nevertheless, the impressibility of other students was of central concern: "The policy of the school committee might well be keyed to a desire on the part of the school committee not to *appear* to condone conduct on the part of unmarried students of a nature to cause pregnancy.... [Hargraves] finds the twelve-to-fourteen age group to be still flexible in their attitudes; they might be led to believe that the school authorities are condoning premarital relations if they were to allow *girl* students in plaintiff's situation to remain in school" (emphases added). Here the intolerant authority of adults who anticipated students' behavior overpowered the evidence of actual students' behaviors and attitudes of accepting their classmate. Comparing this response to my earlier mention of students being hailed as political agents in the wake of school desegregation is telling; the students' sovereignty, maturity, and civic role are not obvious or agreed upon across various contexts and in the eyes of disparate adults—nor are they worth investment. Instead, young people's lack of self-management functions as the basis for justifying codified intolerance.

Stigmatized bodies are always in a complicated relationship with sight because visual conspicuity enables stigmatization at the same time as it erases stigmatized people politically and socially (Garland-Thompson 2002, 56). Stigma, like disability "operates visually by juxtaposing the singular (therefore strange) mark of impairment in a surrounding context of the expected (therefore familiar)," thereby giving meaning to an "impairment" (59–60). Unwed pregnant girls at school threatened to create a new visual narrative of school-age (unwed) pregnancy as tolerable reproduction.

Despite these deterrents, the ultimate *Ordway* ruling established a precedent: by allowing unwed mothers to remain in school, the humanity of young, unwed mothers could be acknowledged in ways it had been discredited before. The reluctance to grant these rights, however, emphasizes just how pervasive the stigmatization of unwed mothers was and the resistance that would be met by those who advocated on behalf of such women. In the words of one researcher: "the issues [of school-age pregnancy] are not simplistic moral ones—pregnancy is not contagious; pregnant girls do not cause other girls to become pregnant—but ones of risk and that the high risks of pregnancy in adolescence deserve the same conscientious objective support and effort toward solution that is made in other areas" (Howard 1971, 364).

Case law, and the context of school-as-politicized space from which it emerged, illustrates tensions about students' bodies and in the processes of gendering that shaped appropriate management of these bodies. School-age people were potentially capable and susceptible beings. In the case of school-age unwed pregnancy, this capability/susceptibility tension ultimately reinforced visibly pregnant women as a primary threat to purity and pure women's susceptibility to corrosive and shameful displays of unrighteous tolerance. Equally likely, those expressing a shared fear of the consequences of the unwed pregnant body as visible in school could have been fearing the unmanageability of those consequences, especially among young people whose liminality in relation to childhood and adulthood rendered them sometimes self-efficacious and sometimes vulnerable. In sum, as *Perry* and *Ordway* demonstrate, much work would need to be done to shift public, unjust ideas of righteous reproduction.

Title IX: The Promise of Inclusion

Ordway v. Hargraves provided a precedent for rulings on school expulsion, but Title IX is the expression of equality that should have brought an end to dismissal based on unwed pregnancy. As part of the Education Amendments of 1972, Congress passed Title IX in order to protect the rights of female students. The law is far-reaching, although most commonly recognized in this historical context for mandating equal rights on the basis of sex to school-sponsored physical fitness and sports programs. Title IX also mandates the protection of women against discrimination in education, a site of coverage not included in the Civil Rights Act of 1964. Pregnant students, in particular, are granted three protections. Title IX forbids schools from denying admission to students on the basis of pregnancy (regardless of marital status), makes unlawful forced separate schooling for pregnant students (a practice that was common at the time), and demands that voluntary segregated classrooms for pregnant students are equal to those for nonpregnant students. In establishing these protections, Title IX likens pregnancy to a temporary medical disability, thus allowing Congress to provide a familiar framework for an otherwise sweeping mandate. This medical disability framework perpetuates students' non-normative status and reaffirms pregnant bodies as the necessary site for protectionist intervention while simultaneously deflecting attention from women's additional identities and needs as school-age mothers-to-be.

Title IX was the product of two sets of congressional hearings, the first being held by US Representative Edith Green in 1970. Hearing testimony explored various practices of sex-based discrimination in higher education. Some administrators openly described a common practice whereby a woman could only be admitted to a college if her grade point average was higher than that considered acceptable for male applicants. This candid response troubled some congresspeople, and the issue of how to end gender-based discrimination "immediately" became a "contentious issue" around the hearings (Department of Education 2003, 14). In subsequent years, five competing bills addressing gender equality in education were drafted. Ultimately, competing bills sponsored by Senators Birch Bayh and George McGovern were combined to create the Title IX legislation that was approved in both houses of Congress before being signed into law by President Richard Nixon in June 1972. The legislation was an antidote to these imbalances in secondary education admissions and addressed concerns over girls' presence and depiction in teaching and learning materials. The three-part mandate for pregnant students, applicable at the secondary level, marked a significant advance in the acknowledgement of and advocacy for unwed pregnant students.

By figuring, without further caveat, pregnancy as analogous to "any other temporary disability," this call for accommodations permits courts of law to interpret its meaning as needed, on a case-by-case basis. Given this disability frame, the text implies that pregnancy does not function as a distinct condition warranting unique accommodations (Brake 2010, 171–72). Rather than a malevolent attempt to label pregnant, school-age girls disabled, the designation is economical and potentially expedient—a shortcut that prevented lawmakers from having to explicate the complex bodily exigences related to school-age pregnancy. Despite its premise of equality, the just spirit of the law is compromised by the crude rhetorical mechanism it employs. Likening pregnancy to a truly temporary disability, such as a broken ankle, suggests that it is a "condition" primarily of the body that precedes recovery. Pregnancy might represent a temporary gestational period, but the resulting delivery does not signal a simple return to predisability conditions. Instead, birthing a child represents the beginning of ongoing physical, emotional, and material transformations for the mother, who, in the early 1970s as I have shown, is still stigmatized for a school-age pregnancy. Thus, the law's rhetoric illuminates the rationalizations and visual premises upon which it is based: that once a student does not look pregnant, her pregnancy is of little relevance to her education or the rights and protections school administrators should guarantee her. Subtly, stigma and impressionability continue to lurk.

Further, the construction of pregnancy as abnormality reflects an idea generally accepted by disability scholars that such categorization enables "the invisible presence of a pure and unmarked center" (Dolmage and Lewiecki-Wilson 2010, 33). In this case, there are three centers: the pure mother (she is not an unmarried student), the pure female student (she is not sexually available), and the pure classroom (in which no visible markers of students' sexuality exist). The visual power of the young, unwed, pregnant body in juxtaposition with the tenaciously guarded, ostensibly asexual space of the classroom can help to explain this tendency in the early 1970s to continue to construct unwed pregnancy as a problem and, in the case of Title IX, as a disability. A medical framing was arguably the most credible framing given that, in this context, school-age pregnant women were feared and thus distrusted. The language of *Perry* and *Ordway* suggests that part of the stigmatization of unwed pregnancy was, historically, the fear that the visible unwed pregnant body within the classroom would imply identification with that body. Thus, meaning-making that follows from "the logic of the visual" (Dolmage and Lewiecki-Wilson 2010, 32) likely informed later, more tolerant but still stigmatizing, constructions of unwed pregnancy and righteous reproduction. A medicalized framing enabled a more credible and stable basis for this legal change by degree—change steeped in the visual politics of shame and within a context where school-age pregnant women were met with fear and distrust.

By understanding school-age pregnant girls as bodies of temporary difference instead of recognizing them as mothers, Title IX indirectly subverts the recognition of such students as humans with rights to dignity and safety as reproducing and/or parenting people. This denial is far less overt than that faced by mothers who anonymously surrendered a child for adoption, but it nevertheless perpetuates a practice of seeing young unwed mothers as problematically pregnant, rather than as people with reproductive sovereignty who can draw from knowledge and experiences of their communities and as mothers in their own right. These bodies are understood as stigmatized, and these legal documents directly and indirectly uphold their stigmatization by defining unwed pregnant students as inherently different than other students. Insofar as the person with a stigma is "by definition . . . not quite human" (Goffman 1963, 5), then discussions of the rights and privileges of unwed students must establish their full humanity in order to compensate from stigma's discrediting power. Because Title IX does not reframe unwed pregnant students in this way, the overall goal of the legislation is compromised.

Indeed, as a law addressing school-age pregnant girls in the 1970s, Title IX failed (and continues to underperform), given the dearth of its de facto implementation (Pillow 2004, 61). In other words, school authorities did (and still do) have the latitude to ultimately determine if and when unwed pregnant students should be forced out of the classroom, which resulted in many girls not experiencing the benefit afforded by the law. Feminist scholar Deborah L. Brake (2010) contends that Title IX employs a "distinctive" legal approach that is "substantive and results oriented," thus allowing the legislation to be especially effective in comparison with other discrimination laws (8). Nevertheless, much like *Brown v. Board of Education*'s decree for schools to desegregate with "all deliberate speed"—language that undercut the potency of this Supreme Court's ruling—Title IX failed to ensure school compliance in terms of protecting pregnant students' rights. Such nonuniform application of the law leads Pillow (2004) to argue that "teen mothers remain the unmentionables and the unknowns" of the amendment (56), suggesting that marked, unwed, pregnant bodies experience residual cultural shame that more "fit" bodies do not. These students' de jure protections, established as early as 1972, were not policed; thus, the de facto convention of denying pregnant students access to school space continued widely. The law functions as a shift from the punishment of deviance to the management of a disability, supplanting critical attention to sexual/gendered injustice with another register of marked difference. Although only an exercise in speculation, one wonders what practices could have emerged with a more robust rhetorical construction of students' educational rights and needs as pregnant people and potentially mothers, rather than disabled bodies that legally should be granted access to the classroom.

"Grotesque" Bodies: Backlash to Tolerance

Even though not a wide social practice, some administrators did permit pregnant students to attend school, even before Title IX went into effect. Such inclusion made the idea of unwed pregnancy within the classroom a reality and prompted a public reckoning of this long-held juxtaposition. One such early attempt at integrating pregnant students into the school environment, that of Citrus High described above, provides a sense of how pregnant girls' access to the mainstream classroom was sometimes met with rhetorics of disgust and revulsion.

It was in early April 1971, about one month after the *Ordway v. Hargraves* ruling, when Judy Fay—a white honor student like Fay Ordway—was *Life*'s cover story. Citrus High had a far more understanding relationship with its students than did Middlesex High, the administration encouraging girls to stay in school until the last two weeks of their pregnancy and return to school with their babies six weeks after giving birth, taking a combination of home economics, child care, and "standard academic" courses (Woodbury 1971, 35). Principal James Georgeou developed the program based on his belief that teenage pregnancy should be treated "'not as a social disease but as a fact of life'" (38). Georgeou met resistance from the Citrus school board, but the school's "spirit of incentive" resulted in many of the maternity program girls graduating early. Fay serves as an example of the benefit of the program because her "heavy [post-pregnancy] course load . . . will enable her to graduate in June" and then go to college, "something she hadn't even considered before she got pregnant" (40).

Citrus's program seems to have functioned as a well-developed version of earlier experiments in specialized education for unwed pregnant girls, such as that tested at Webster School in Washington, DC, as early as 1963. The Webster School, however, focused primarily on the needs of Black students and thus would not have necessarily disrupted white conventions that linked whiteness to sexual purity and the alleged benefits of sexualized shame. Significantly, the Webster School and its students also never made the cover of *Life* magazine. The lead story suggests that the trend of allowing white, school-age pregnant girls in school was beginning to take hold even as it portrays Citrus in near-utopian terms. The benefit of allowing pregnant girls to remain in school seems to reverse the effects of impressibility so feared by other administrators, for as the article notes, "now that there are pregnant girls at Citrus, the boys have cleaned up their language, courteously hold open doors and even push strollers" (Woodbury 1971, 40). The article—and various pictures of Fay and other pregnant students comfortably interacting with other students, teachers, and administrators—provides narrative and visual proof that at Citrus, unwed pregnant bodies do not function as reminders of a problem that should be erased, but rather as correctives to the immaturity and self-absorption of adolescence. At the same time, the article perpetuates a long-held, often citizen-oriented, attribution of US mothers as being morally suasive agents responsible for the boys and men in their lives—the effects of which were thought to support nation-building goals in the early republic (Robbins 2004) and even now, in the twenty-first century US security state (Fixmer-Oraiz 2019). As a call for inclusion, the profile implicitly demonstrates Fay's presence as upholding (racially coded white) "harmony" as Vinson suggests and as mitigating and managing a menacing unmanageability of school-age bodies that were imagined to be vulnerable to viral libidinous impressibility in the absence of moralizing shame.

The move to grant unmarried pregnant girls access to the classroom was one for which many Americans were not ready, if the responses to *Life*'s feature is any indication. Reader J. A. Siegel (1971) laments in a subsequent issue that the "cover sets some sort of a new dimension of achievement in crass, lurid, inelegant journalistic bad taste. To proffer a picture of this pathetic schoolchild with her grotesque maternity figure over the bold-type title "High School Pregnancy" simply makes a bad, sad, scene" (20A). Save one response from Principal Georgeou, all of the letters to the editor disparaged *Life*'s decision to report on the story of the girls and school programs described by the piece. Readers did not appreciate the magazine's suggestion that "life" now included accepting pregnant girls into school spaces and supporting them as they balanced obtaining an education and preparing to have a baby.

Siegel's comments critique the *visibility* of Fay's body on the cover of the magazine, making apparent the letter writer's own beliefs: that such errant (white) bodies should remain hidden from public view and that evidence of these bodies, such as publicized pictures and magazine articles, violates righteousness. That the magazine would make the story of this unwed pregnant student its feature and go so far as to put her "grotesque" body on the cover offends Siegel's stigmaphobic sensibilities. The visual rhetorical power of Judy Fay's body overrides the ability for Siegel, like so many others, to reframe unwed pregnancy as Principal Georgeou did, as a natural "fact of life" rather than a "social disease," a term that implies fears of infectious unrighteousness and the racial and status-based connotations that can so easily stick to such a figuration. Siegel's comments convey revulsion and less overtly suggest that Fay's presence—on the magazine's cover and in the normalized space of the high school classroom—intrudes upon what should be stigmaphobic space, threatening to render it stigmaphilic as a public site of education, dignity, safety, and tolerance.

Compromised Rhetorics of Justice

As public discussion slowly started to address the need to replace racialized and patriarchal practices of hiding some unwed pregnant women with more strategic and just measures for addressing the putative repercussions of a "new permissiveness," those needing protection from stigmatized, unwed, pregnant bodies changed. In relation to young women, "protections" varied across communities and locations. Public knowledge of sterilization abuse by the early 1970s revealed that non-white youth were preventatively adultified, denied identities of innocence, and deemed unrighteous reproducers because of anticipatory beliefs of their unmanaged, and thus ominously unmanageable fertility futures. As equal protections based on sex became a legal mandate, the vestiges of a logic of protecting school spaces and the student bodies in them became apparent. The irony here resides in that the very discussions about unwed pregnancy that perpetuated these latter shifts were discussions about the students' own protections as individuals with rights and liberties just like others their age.

The bodies of young, "school-age" people were, in the 1970s, frequently deemed real threats to be responsively managed or anticipated threats to be preemptively managed. In both cases, they were considered dangers to the patriarchal, raced, and sexually righteous normalcy of the high school classroom or to the United States more generally. The danger of "school-age pregnancy" in this recent historical moment, then, perpetuated and was perpetuated by public discursive "narrative scripts" that rendered young women's bodies a public site for intervention, regulation, and in some cases violence. Law and literature scholar Karla FC Holloway (2011) argues that such public narratives "very nearly dismiss the private" (15). The visual symbolism of unwed pregnancy reduced young, unwed, mothers-to-be to distended bellies that could provoke the fears of contagion, larger threats of race mixing as one aspect of unmitigated desire, as well as the need to intervene on behalf of the disabled, in/valid body. Thus, unwed pregnant girls functioned as a highly visible, social identity based on difference that enabled processes of stigmatization, even at a time of (in the context of public education) increasing legal affordances. According to Holloway, this move toward public presence and tolerance warrants scrutiny because "Identity matters when private personhood is made public. In a public sphere, where gender or race reign through the force of social construct, historical pattern, and even constitutional authority, social narratives are shaped within the nation's body politic. . . . There are some bodies that will and can ordinarily disappear into the normative, that are not vulnerable to the socialized identity scripts that ensnare public narratives" (14). School-age pregnant women of the early 1970s as well as young women who were anticipated to most likely use their sexual and reproductive capabilities in unsanctioned ways were subject to management through mechanisms that continued to rely on logics of gendered shame and stigma. These same people—as I will go on to show in this book—would be the focus of ensuing public narratives calling for further social management of their young, potentially reproducing bodies.

A slowly emerging public issue in the early 1970s, unwed pregnancy functioned less as a symbol of private, familial shame and more as a complex problem that was rhetorically incompatible with the goals of education, while socially and morally incongruous with the notion of the US high school as a place of supposed normativity, obedience, and lack of desire. According to Martha Nussbaum (2004), the "desire to stigmatize [cannot be] a rational basis for law" (271), thus suggesting the compromised affordances for true human rights and justice in this historical context. This finding calls attention to the incongruity of an emotion like shame, with its reliance on some integrity/dishonor continuum (a concept I return to in the conclusion), and of rational efforts to secure rights and assure justice in a noncontingent manner. Despite claims of a pervasive, new, sexual permissiveness, some women—including very young women—were, in this moment, forever denied the right to have a child because of their social location. Additionally, the custom of denying pregnant girls' access to this school space continued, unlawfully, demonstrating a continued social adherence to shaming and punishing girls (primarily, if not exclusively) for sexual impropriety. In short, shame, now operationalized more publicly and structurally through stigmatizing rhetorics, was not washed away by a new, culturally sanctioned, sexual permissiveness. Instead, unwed pregnant bodies in public elicited clearer expressions of lingering shame that was mapped onto women's visibly different, or anticipatorily unrighteous, bodies.

Three

Macrochange, Reproductive Agency, and the Stickiness of Shame

I n 2010, Patti Hawn (sister of actress Goldie Hawn) published *Good Girls Don't,* a memoir of being a pregnant white teenager in the 1950s. Hawn later commented on the importance of sharing her story:

> *Good Girls Don't* is about an era on the eve of the sexual revolution, prior to *Roe vs. Wade,* when many women died from illegal abortions. It is a unique time in history, foreign to an entire generation of women. . . . My book is a deeply personal first-hand account of what it was like to be held captive in an unwanted pregnancy at the close of an era where home economics took precedence over sex education. It tells the story of the last generation of young women to experience life on the eve of the sexual revolution and the decisions a young woman makes based on this early trauma. (quoted in Sharples 2016)

Whether familiar with the stories of "girls in trouble" or not, Hawn's readers likely would not question her assertion that the era of going away had come to a close by 1973, when the US Supreme Court decriminalized abortion. Of the scant histories of this experience, most prominently situate the 1973 *Roe v. Wade* ruling as the primary marker of a cultural shift away from the hiding, secrets, and shame of unwed pregnancy that was so common through the 1960s (Fessler 2007; Glaser 2020; Solinger 2000). Similarly, in writing that draws upon her personal experiences, rhetoric and composition scholar Nancy Welch also points to *Roe* and its immediately preceding case law to emphasize the changing landscape of women's reproduction in the 1970s. Welch explains that these "landmark decisions" both "liberalized access to birth control information and devices" and "extended the protections of privacy to (some) sexual practices and decisions" (18). There is no doubt that *Roe* effected significant change, both in relation to the spirit and the letter of the law. But what did this time of legal and technological change mean for unmarried women who were having sex and/or becoming pregnant? And how did these changes address or fail to address the sexual and reproductive realities of other marginalized women?

I consider these questions in light of two reasons that historically circulated to explain the perceived ebb of righteous shame culture and, subsequently, fewer instances of hiding an "illicit" pregnancy: (1) the development of the birth control pill and (2) women's increased access to abortion after the *Roe* ruling. (The third cause—a purported new sexual permissiveness—is the focus of the previous chapter.) As the last chapter made clear, by the early 1970s fewer white women were "going away" to secret an unwed pregnancy. As I argue throughout this book, however, shame endures and does not easily dissolve. Rhetorical shaming and stigmatization of unwed pregnant bodies (especially white bodies) continued past the 1960s, even when legislation was passed to make public institutions—like high schools—open and accessible to unwed pregnant students. Similarly, throughout the 1970s, at a time of public and flourishing white feminist consciousness, shame's interconnectedness to womanhood across communities lingered, emerging in new ways and as a site of consciousness-raising and public reflection. Shame's persistence can be traced within the histories of these technological and legislative/juridical changes as well as through various ways that activists and artists reckon with new relationships to gender, sexuality, and reproductive health.

This chapter interrogates two sites of macrochange—the development of the pill and the *Roe* decision—as viable explanations for why white women supposedly no longer had to hide their unwed pregnancy. I also link and analyze sites of microchange—varied texts about women's sexual and reproductive lives that were created, circulated within, and contributed to this historical moment. To explain shame's mutability and evidence its endurance, I consider the visible politics and affective dispositions of shame across these macro and micro sites, interrogating how shame—an affect communicated, perceived, and/or felt—contributed to an affective rhetorical ecology of ongoing righteousness. Within this new ecology, I investigate which bodies could be openly desirous, whose pregnancy or reproductive lives could be acknowledged and supported publicly, and how this publicity figured various affective responses.

Such historiographic work can always reveal, in the words of theorist Kenneth Burke (1962), a selection of reality, a reflection of reality, and therefore a deflection of reality (59). I leverage this Burkean method to suggest what a public focus on the pill and *Roe* reflects about recovery narratives of righteous reproduction and to attend to what these explanations continue to deflect. To wit, narratives that link the decline of shame—shame that must be understood as an aspect of righteous reproduction as a raced, classed, and historically specific construct—with the selected macrochanges of women's access to the birth control pill and to abortion through decriminalization based on the *Roe* decision reflect anxieties about the radicalness of women's possible and positive sexual and reproductive sovereignty. Likewise, a shame-oriented declension narrative indexes the power of women's sexual liberation—a genie of sexual and reproductive control that could not be put back in its bottle and that therefore signaled the threat (or promise) of movement into personal, social, and cultural unknowns.[1]

Simultaneously, the pervasive narrative of "women's" liberation through legal and technological means is a problematic deflection in three ways. First, narratives of macrochange uphold a fiction of a dissipation of gendered shame that runs counter to ongoing and even contemporary experiences of the presence of gendered—and especially sexual—shame and shaming. Simply put, many people continue to feel and experience the effects of shame's relationship to gendered subordination and relationships among sexuality, righteousness, power, and violence, which is the reason that shame remains a "topic with deep and persistent significance for feminists" (Fischer 2018, 372). Such publicly galvanizing macrosites of change in medicine and law offer a vital opportunity for rhetorical historiographic revision and more nuanced understandings of *how* shame endures.

Second, broad public allegiance to narratives of macrochange overlook key experiences, including women's complicated and uneven uptake of reproductive control, the partiality of such change across experiences and communities, and even the political reversal of the affordances of greater fertility management among poor and often doubly marginalized women by the late 1970s. More complete historiography does the justice-oriented work of linking upstream and downstream parts of these macronarratives: the development of the pill, the norms-based case law that served as the precedent to *Roe*'s protection of privacy, and the passage of the Hyde Amendment that limited abortion access and created an aperture for new forms of righteous public shaming of reproducing people. Further, linking cross-community perspectives illuminates how less righteous women (e.g., unwed women, poor women, women in US territories who ingested medicine-in-development) contributed to processes of change that would disrupt and reconfigure righteous reproduction and various forms of reproductive and sexual possibility. Additionally linking sites of macrochange to sites of microchange offers a more robust sense of shame as a persistent political and public emotion during this time.

Third, I focus throughout the chapter on the publicity of these sites of change by considering how they reflect reproductive justice's critique of the incompleteness of sexual autonomy based on the negative rights of privacy, which translates in the United States as a freedom from state intervention into matters of reproductive control. This model fails to support affirmative freedoms to act with sovereignty and enjoy sex and reproduction as a comprehensive human right based in dignity and safety for all people. It also enables such negative freedoms to be upheld, modified, or revoked by legislative regimes possibly bolstering partisan public will. As an opportunity based on an affirmative, human rights orientation, true macrochange as reproductive justice would be a fully public concern that warrants public understanding and tolerance, related public support (through social policy and commensurate funding/access), and public trust in people to make appropriate decisions about sex and reproduction for themselves with such understanding and support in place. In addition to contributing to a reproductive justice critique of the limitations of grand narratives of "choice" as an agential gain, I offer the concept of affective realignment in my examination of microsites of change to shed light on how various people's ideas about sovereignty and sexual freedom from this same era of macrochange evidence a pastiche of shame-resistant approaches that, together, provide more durable and affirmative possibilities.

In short, changes related to unrighteous pregnancy during the volatile 1970s are best understood by examining the interstices among technological developments, nonexpert discourses relating to women's sexual health and behavior, court rulings (codified, rationalized decisions made on behalf of the people in the United States), and the unarticulated subtexts of these decisions. By sharing this context, I demonstrate that macrochange narratives overemphasize and erroneously imply the universality of women's reproductive agency and that they depict change as affording agency in problematic and untenable ways—as a salubrious gift given to women through scientific and legislative channels. My critique of agency-as-granted by the pill and *Roe* suggests that without such historiographic interventions, the macronarratives explaining how mid-century architectures of shame and silence began to shift will continue to capitulate to the power of patriarchal and supremacist institutions. Narratives that fail to lay bare the sticky rhetorics of persistent shame that are part of this moment of profound change continue to silence the nonhierarchical and collective rhetorical avenues by which women cultivated sexual sovereignty and reconfigured themselves away from the long reach of entrenched and publicly circulating ideas and feminized effects of gendered shame. By recovering these alternative sites of affective realignment and placing them alongside a more fully inclusive retelling of medical and judicial advancement, I offer a historiographic intervention to support more ambiguous, skeptical, and biopolitically attuned understandings of gendered sexual and reproductive agency and sovereignty.

Macrochange 1: The Pill as Innovation

Early support for the development of a birth control pill came from activist and nurse Margaret Sanger as well as Katharine Dexter McCormick, a monied and well-educated woman who, like Sanger, was dedicated to pursuing effective and accessible methods for women to manage their own fertility. The two women met in the early part of the century, but it was not until 1950 that McCormick sought Sanger's help in locating a researcher who she could sponsor to develop birth control technology. McCormick's willingness to fund such investigation cannot be overemphasized, for oral contraceptive research was considered inappropriate by the pharmaceutical industry and government-backed researchers (May 2010, 22). Gregory Pincus was just the type of researcher Sanger and McCormick were pursuing, and after connecting with the benefactors, he collaborated with John Rock to develop a hormonal pill that would prevent the release of a fertilizable egg and subsequently prevent conception.

Pincus and Rock conducted extensive clinical trials of the drug in Puerto Rico in 1956, thereby dodging US laws prohibiting contraception use in order to test the pill's efficacy (May 2010, 29). Once this research proved successful in terms of the researchers' goals, pharmaceutical company G.D. Searle began supplying Enovid in 1957. As the nation's first contraception pill, Enovid was marketed as a treatment for menstrual disorders and infertility. Two years later Searle applied to the Food and Drug Administration (FDA) for approval of the pill as a form of contraception, which was granted in 1960. The FDA insisted that approval was based only on the safety of the pill, not on the political or moral implications of its use (Gibbs 2010, 43; May 2010, 32–33).

Testing of the oral contraceptive is one aspect of pill development that must be recognized as an integral part of the ethically unsound and raced practices of this "innovation." Puerto Rico offered a perfect blend of networked clinics, capable physicians able to organize and deploy contraceptive trials, and a population of women eager to participate. At the same time, an anti-sex bias in the United States discouraged researchers from testing a technology that would potentially separate sexual activity from procreation (Schoen 2005, 208–12). Many Puerto Rican women were desperately wanting to control their own fertility, and some of the participants in the contraception testing failed to qualify for elective sterilization procedures on the basis of age and current number of children. Fears of overpopulation among poor people created a precipitating context for taking the trials to Puerto Rico and conducting them in an unethical and rigorous fashion (Briggs 2003, 136–37). While early efforts to test among more well-educated Puerto Rican women were both taxing on participants and relatively ineffectual, later trials targeting poorer Puerto Rican women that asked for less active participation provided a larger participant group (López 2008, 17; Schoen 2005, 210–11).

Many researchers (and Pincus in particular) flatly ignored the complaints women expressed during these trials about the side effects of taking the pill; at this time, regulation of human subjects was poor even if some researchers and doctors (Rock, for instance) *were* concerned about the tangential harm of taking the drug (Briggs 2003, 134; Schoen 2005, 212). Various side effects—harbingers of later critiques of hormonal contraception raised by US women's health movement activists—were reported by the Puerto Rican women who ingested the test drug. In any case, many poor women in the territory—850 by 1958—faced a high-risk testing environment in which their bodies and their health became the basis for registering the effectiveness of an experimental drug. McCormick's call for a "cage of ovulating females" (whether Puerto Rican or from a population of residential patients in a mental health facility in Massachusetts—another set of subjects) sheds light on the inhumane aspects of such technological development that would go on to bring "liberation" to many white women in the United States (quoted in Briggs 2003, 135). And while Puerto Rican physicians such as Edris Rice-Wray and Penny Satterthwaite ostensibly used the trials in part to leverage trial participation into an opportunity for providing other health care services to women who did not otherwise have such access (Schoen 2005, 212–13), the feminist implications of the development of the pill are murky at best. Briggs persuasively argues for holding "women and feminists"—Sanger, McCormick, but also other medical and social professionals in Puerto Rico—most accountable for acting in solidarity to exert such colonial violence on non-white women, largely in the name of lowering unmitigated population rates among poor people (Briggs 2003, 137–39).

In short, while the blame for undesirable trials can be challenging to assign, the complicated and power-laden history of pill development needs to be an essential part of any discussion of contraception as an avenue for "women's" agency. As Schoen explains, Puerto Rican women did not have access to "decent reproductive care," and this fact is an essential aspect of the conditions for the trials being developed and for the participants who served as bodyminds who enabled the trials to proceed. Participants traded access to some reproductive control for the assurances of a safe and effective experience taking the pill—a tradeoff that "might have met physicians and women's short-term interests but left larger structural problems of health care access unsolved" (Schoen 2005, 213).

Any recounting of the history of the oral contraceptive must also grapple with how the technology is tied up with its unjust and violent applications in the posttrial phase. In her sweeping and public-facing history of Black-focused medical experimentation in the United States, Harriet A. Washington (2008) describes Sanger as "the most famous American popularizer of eugenics" while also noting that she is most typically praised for her roles as a feminist and as a key figure in the development of birth control.[2] "All these labels fit," Washington contends (195). Washington explains that in 1939, Sanger created the Negro Project as a response to Black women's lack of access to health care. She writes that in creating "experimental 'family planning centers,'" the Negro Project enabled Sanger to devise a strategy to "find the best way of reducing the black population by promoting eugenic principles" (197). Washington further connects this "experiment of addressing black social ills with the application of negative eugenics via black birth control clinics" directly to the later opening of Planned Parenthood clinics in "central urban areas" (198). While it is true that Sanger championed the freedom of "women" through the ability for them to have control of their bodies, birth control must be remembered as a divisive topic, material, and practice that functioned simultaneously as a "eugenic prescription" and as a "matter of private decision making" (Solinger 2007, 101). Additionally, Dorothy Roberts (2017) reminds that eugenics language imparted to Sanger's audiences a level of scientific credibility suggesting that the birth control movement was a matter of public health and national welfare concern (72).

When considering historiography related to oral contraception and those who facilitated its development and access, one must grapple with the vexed role that such technology has assumed across white and non-white communities, across affluent and poor communities, and between women and men within these various communities. While Black Nationalists famously criticized and resisted Black women's use of contraception because of the belief that it was being deployed as a form of targeted population control, Black activist women were not necessarily in agreement. For instance, the Black Women's Liberation Group of Mount Vernon, New York (a group comprised mostly of poor and working-class people) centered women's control of their own fertility as part of a wider platform of women's liberation and a vision of women's leadership in Black liberation efforts (Nelson 2003, 61). They put these ideas in their 1968 "Statement on Birth Control," which was addressed to Black men. At the same moment, Frances Beal, an organizer for the Student Nonviolent Coordinating Committee's Black Women's Liberation Committee similarly resisted sexism apparent in the Black liberation movement. This resistance countered movement participants' acceptance of the myth of Black matriarchy as expressed by Daniel Patrick Moynihan several years earlier (62).

The voices of activist leaders reflect conflicting dynamics of race, gender, and class; at the same time, research conducted just several years later substantiated the presence of deep fears about the uses of new contraceptive technologies among Black communities. For instance, a 1973 survey published in the *American Journal of Public Health* (AJPH) reported that "genocidal fears are widely held in the black population" and "that 39% of the entire sample [of 1,890 people] believed that 'birth control programs are a plot to eliminate blacks'"—which the researchers assessed was an "ample basis for distress" (Turner and Darity 1973, 1033). Another study (by the same authors and also published in

AJPH) confirmed that by the early 1970s, there was an increase in media coverage that questioned a link between race genocide and family planning programs, further evidencing the perception of a real government-sponsored plot to limit Black reproduction (Darity and Turner 1972, 1455). The distrust felt by some Black women and the uncomfortable reckoning some women had when taking birth control is part of the historical and affective story of oral contraceptive use. It is also one of several reasons why reproductive justice advocates have long called for an eschewal of a "choice" paradigm when discussing reproductive issues. The perspective of one Black social worker in 1966 explains this conundrum: "Negroes don't want children they can't take care of, but we are afraid to trust you [white people] when your offered help has so often turned out to be exploitation" (quoted in Caron 1998, 550).

During the 1960s, the pill as a prophylactic form of social medicine undeniably became the hope for controlling population growth and lowering abortion rates. Use of the pill, however, was varied among women and simply did not meet supporters' high expectations for quick and sweeping change. The race-based ideal of white women's sexual purity discouraged some such women from wanting to take an oral contraceptive because this would signal that they were preparing to—and thus, problematically, wanting to—have sex, an especially risky proposition outside of marriage. Catholics, particularly married couples, were eager to use the pill as a form of birth control, because of the rationale that, as a hormonal method for extending the "safe" window for having sex according to the rhythm method, it fell outside the Catholic Church's ban on contraception. But in 1968, Pope Paul issued an encyclical, *Humanae Vitae*, banning the use of any artificial birth control and leaving many Catholics using the pill discouraged, if not disaffected (May 2010, 124–25). Further, married couples were not legally permitted to obtain contraception until 1965, and only after a Supreme Court ruling; it would be years later that legal protection would extend to unmarried women. Additionally, the pill (and the IUD, also available in 1960) posed so many health concerns that both were generally considered unsafe until the 1970s. And if all of these complications were not enough, women had to get a prescription for the pill from a doctor (like they would an IUD or a diaphragm); many unmarried women—whether borrowing a wedding ring to pose as a married woman or not—may well have experienced shame in making this request (Fessler 2007, 43).

Early advertising from pharmaceutical companies to physicians reflect the patronizing and patriarchal contexts in which physicians and husbands acted as gatekeepers and surveillors of women, figured as incompetent and unreliable, who were now technologically enabled to control their own fertility management.[3] These advertisements reflect rhetorical efforts to affirm the need for male domination over hapless women, thus suggesting anxieties over the autonomy (sexual and otherwise) that pill use could afford. When understood as windows into this moment of change, these texts make apparent what was likely a more ambiguous and complicated moment for those women open to the idea of pill use. In her foundational theorizing on shame as a gendered emotion, Sandra Lee Bartky (1990) calls attention to such moments of ambiguity —situations "affirming women in some ways and diminishing them in others" as central to the subtle, persistent, and entirely public ways that gendered shame is communicated (94). The corrosive result is "not so much a belief as a *feeling* of inferiority or a *sense* of inadequacy" (94; emphasis in original); accordingly, such suasive messages as historiographic markers of dispositions and attunements are a useful supplement to this narrative of technological and medical macrochange.

Despite the thorny discussions of development, access, and safety described above, the pill was used more widely in the 1970s than in the 1960s. But as women increasingly gained more control of their fertility, use of this technology aligned with fears of rampant levels of "venereal disease" (a now-antiquated term for sexually transmitted infections, or STIs). Earlier, in the 1950s, venereal infections were thought to have lessened enough to be at most a minor public health threat (Brandt 1985, 171). STIs were of ongoing concern for many years, often considered a scourge carried by unrighteous US and "foreign" women, infecting military personnel on duty at alarming rates. But research advances in penicillin provided a sense of false reassurance by mid-century that venereal infections, especially syphilis and gonorrhea, were easily curable (Lord 2010, 71–92).

The end of STIs, however, was not in sight, and rates of "venereal disease" were on the rise. Public health officials attributed a spike in STIs to what they dubbed the "three p's": permissiveness, promiscuity, and the pill (Parascandola 2008, 138). Even though this explanation suggested that rates of infections rose because of the late-1960s sexual revolution, cases of infection actually tripled as early as 1957, an entire decade before San Francisco's summer of love (Lord 2010, 116). By 1972, a national commission claimed that rates of STIs had reached epidemic proportions (Parascandola 2008, 141). And by 1975, gonorrhea and syphilis were, respectively, the first and third most prevalent communicable diseases in the United States (Brandt 1985, 175). These high STI rates demonstrated to the public that there was no magic solution after all, and the discovery of the incurable Herpes Simplex II in 1979 was touted as a "sexual leprosy" to be feared (Allyn 2001, 292).

Historians speculate that the increasing spread of STIs is directly linked to waning government funds allocated for disease research, as well as to public health education efforts that were thwarted by a conservative social climate that devalued sexual literacy. Nevertheless, there was a perception that women's sexual freedom was the largest contributing factor of this rise (Lord 2010, 124–27). Specifically, such infections functioned as "proof" of "revelatrice infidelity" or sexual looseness (Brandt 1985, 180). So as the pill became more available and allowed women and men to have sex increasingly "free" of the "hassle" of other birth control technologies (such as condoms), women became more exposed to these infections and simultaneously became "responsible" for carrying them in yet another iteration of a misogynistic trope.

Despite the pill's complicated history, it continues to elicit magic-bullet narratives of instant and sweeping change, especially in documentaries that perpetuate tropes of "women's" full and unfettered ability to be in control of their fertility, their ability to replace worry (of unintended pregnancy) with reassurance, and their burgeoning ability to cultivate a relationship with desire. Similarly, a 1966 *Saturday Evening Post* article proclaimed that a "birth control revolution" promised "the American woman, already the freest in the world, still vaster freedom" (Nillson and Spencer 2015). However, the same article warns that the development of the pill means freedom that, "extends not only to wives but to unmarried girls, and the choices that the latter make can mean a widening of the rift between the generations." The complex emotional responses to women as pill users as felt by women themselves is only part of the affective context of this moment. Fear of unmonitored, unmanaged, and unrighteous use was also a circulating concern. A telling anecdote from the article calls attention to anxieties related to such freedom when applied unrighteously—when "whether by legitimate or underground routes, the pill has found its way to the college campuses and even to the high-school hallways":

> Dr. Mary Steichen Calderone, an eminent planned-parenthood expert, tells of an encounter with a girl in a New York City junior high school during a break between classes. The girl had dropped her handbag in the crowded corridor, and its contents spilled on the floor. "I stopped to help her pick the things up," Doctor Calderone said, "and was astonished to see a package of birth-control pills. I asked the child, 'Do you really know about these things?' 'Oh, yes,' she replied, 'I take them every Saturday night when I go on a date.' She had gotten the pills from her married sister—apparently without benefit of instructions. If it weren't so funny, it would be tragic.' In fact, it probably will be tragic. One pill alone is quite ineffective. They must be taken daily for five to seven days before any protection is built up. (Nillson and Spencer 2015)

What is the generational "rift" the article suggests, and why does a young woman misusing the pill feature in this story of contraceptive "revolution" in 1966? Or, posed differently: what is now to be guarded against—what is to be feared—and why? The fumbling girl—portrayed as physically awkward and cloddish in relation to pill use that nevertheless needs to be explained to the reader—signals the risks of freedom and serves as an anticipatory figure for an ensuing tragedy of unrighteous reproduction. Her ignorance is a foil rather than an invitation for knowledge cultivation about oral prophylactics—a new and thus reasonably unfamiliar form of medicine. Such "liberated" reproduction had not been publicly sanctioned before the pill but now ostensibly was, suggests the article, despite this foreboding story.

Here I consider Ahmed's (2004) broad claim that emotions involve "affective forms of reorientation" and that we can attend to orientations by examining how bodies and objects come into contact (8). Specifically, Ahmed writes that fear "shapes the surfaces of bodies in relation to objects" as a process of this contact (8); Ahmed uses this orientation and contact framework to replace a more typical tendency for reading objects themselves as being inherent sources of fear. Using an example of a child being afraid when coming into contact with a bear, Ahmed argues that any sense that the bear is in fact a fearsome animal is actually an "image that is shaped by cultural histories and memories"—one that nevertheless can register impressionistically as a feeling "on the surface of the skin" despite it being a mediated affect (7). The fear invoked in the story of the high schooler prompts fear of the woman as an unreliable pill user as well as a person potentially emboldened to explore new, more affirmative orientations to sex. The fear of women's agentic possibility is not inherent in the woman or in her contact with the revolutionary pill. Instead, it is a persistent fear that is shaped by deeply misogynistic "cultural histories and memories" wherein few women have been trusted or considered capable of knowing their own bodies.

Additionally, a cultural fascination with the pill-as-miracle-drug obscures the lived experiences and constraints of many women. More than ten years after FDA approval of oral contraceptives, some sexually active women were still in the dark about the fundamentals of sex and conception, much less contraception. Pam, a white woman I interviewed for this project, went to a DePaul home for unwed mothers near Cleveland, Ohio and gave birth during her senior year of high school in 1972. Pam admits that contraception of any kind was not a familiar concept to her. "You know what, to be honest, nobody, it wasn't talked about a lot. We just kind of had to learn about it on our own. Did I know about the Pill? Afterward I sure did! But, um, no. I don't know if I knew about the Pill or not. And protection and stuff? I'm like where was my mind? You know what I mean? I didn't have a lot of information—I didn't. Even in schools back then they didn't educate you about it." Pam's experience illuminates how pervasive silences about sexual lives persisted in the shadow of the sexual revolution, suggesting the vital need for self-knowledge and women's sexual and reproductive advocacy at this time. Pam's willingness to blame herself for this lack of information ("where was my mind?") points to the extent to which women's sense of accountability for sexual literacy to which they had no access could and can be internalized. This internalization is interwoven into larger ambient rhetorical workings of sticky, persistent gendered shame related to women, sex, and reproduction.

While pill development and emergence is remembered in connection to broader social changes at this moment of US history, movement often reflects a modification-by-degree of the status quo guided by the ongoing interests of power holders rather than a deep reversal in ways of thinking to account for perspectives of those who hold less power. When change relates to women's ability to have sovereignty over their bodies, such movement-by-degree can be unjust. Amy Koerber (2018) traces similar scientific and medical movement through time as demonstrating strategic "configurations in which the female mind and body repeatedly emerge as foreign, mysterious, or defective versions of the male mind and body" ("From Hysteria" 186). Further, moments of technological discovery as emergence, when viewed as instances of Koerber's rhetorical (re)configuration, interlink with longer cultural histories of not trusting women to manage their fertility, of not viewing women as capable agents of their lives, in which sexuality and reproduction are a critical part.

For instance, Diedre Cooper Owens (2017) recovers a contrasting history of violence on dehumanized women that sheds light on medical racism, technological discovery, and mercenary decisions to entrust women at strategic moments. Owens argues that nineteenth century Black and Irish immigrant women who were otherwise considered subhuman were violated by white, male medical authorities without consent for the purpose of gynecological research that would benefit white women. Conversely, these same poor and/or enslaved women were later enlisted to provide gynecological care when their labor and expertise was critically needed by the so-called "father of modern gynecology," James Marion Sims. Owens thus illuminates a history in which women were acted upon until they were enlisted as trustworthy actors necessary for maintaining medical credibility and practice. Historically, women have not been deemed capable of or entrusted with body knowledge until such trust is sanctioned by power holders, often for their own interests or within their own parameters of acceptability.

To be sure, the development of the pill as a form of contraception represents a formidable portion of women's reproductive history. But women's ability to assume more control over their own sexuality and sexual behavior was not as ubiquitous, smooth, or affectively liberating as such narratives tend to suggest. The pill produced its own set of complications for sexually active women across communities and contributed to larger and longer histories of mistrust. Popular understandings of the pill, then, construct a potential that the technology could not and did not live up to, no matter how significant its creation was to women's material realities and self-perceptions. The same narrative overextension can be observed, I suggest, in relation to the decriminalization of abortion.

Macrochange 2: *Roe* as Legislated Agency

Although the letter of the law made abortion illegal in the United States for more than 100 years, there was great tolerance for the not-so-secret practice of abortion for much of the twentieth century. Historically, the public acknowledgement of or surreptitious practice of legal or illegal abortion has had little to do with women's agency or autonomy. Instead, abortion was a matter for women and their local networks of care, quietly tolerated—unregulated though illegal—during periods of social rest. It was less tolerated during times when groups of women explicitly sought political power or sexual freedom (e.g., during the first and second "waves" of feminist activism).

For many years—from colonial times through the early nineteenth century —reproductive control was simply not a legal or medical concern. In fact, most Americans found abortion before quickening (the first sign of fetal movement) to be acceptable and nonmoral. During the nineteenth century, however, abortion became a medical issue, an area of purported expertise over which physicians—a group that was gaining professional status—could claim technical knowledge (Luker 1984, 27–35). Medical oversight exerted pressure on unskilled practitioners, many of whom were women, to stop performing abortions and also functioned as a nativist response to the low birthrate among US-born, white women (Allyn 2001, 260). Thus, as abortions increasingly became the province of medicine, doctors adopted the role of custodians who could determine when abortions were justifiable. Women, conversely, were increasingly considered insufficiently able to decide when an abortion was necessary and appropriate because they lacked medical knowledge and were thought to be able to make such a decision only on subjective (here meaning incompetent) grounds (Luker 1984, 44).

By the end of the nineteenth century, as women agitated for suffrage and the United States welcomed an unprecedented number of immigrants to its shores, nearly every state had declared abortion illegal except when needed to save a mother's life, in which case the procedure had to be performed by a physician (Allyn 2001, 261; Caron 2008). Although the medical profession continued to regulate abortion within its own ranks through much of the early twentieth century, by the 1940s and 1950s, doctors were being pressured to more closely follow state laws defining legal abortions (Caron 2008). Simultaneously, hospital abortion boards were established to regulate who could receive "therapeutic abortions" (those performed, legally, by a physician), drastically reducing the number of women who were able to obtain an abortion through these means (Luker 1984, 45–48; Solinger 1998, xi).

During the first half of the twentieth century, there was not significant, mobilized resistance to this stringent approach to granting abortions (Luker 1984, 48). There were, however, an estimated 1.3 million illegal, often dangerous, abortions that took place at this time (Solinger 1998, xi). Additionally, Kristin Luker (1984) explains that it is impossible to know the exact motives for women seeking illegal abortions. Perhaps they did so because they did not anticipate receiving help from a physician, because they requested an abortion and were rejected, or because they were simply fearful or ashamed of raising (or unwilling to raise) the topic in the first place (52). The repression of abortion left all women with little-to-no straightforward information about the procedure, many women with insufficient money or funds to access a "safe" (i.e., legal and/or not life-threatening) abortion, and few women (those who could afford to travel abroad or find a willing abortionist closer to home) with only a hope that they were in qualified hands. Although there are examples of women being arrested for obtaining an illegal abortion, unauthorized providers were more likely to be apprehended. As Rickie Solinger (2007) explains, "the old agreement" of local officials overlooking the presence of abortion was "rather suddenly canceled" even when these procedures showed no evidence of harm being done to women. Sensational coverage of police raids, arrests, and subsequent trials, however, functioned to criminalize this previously everyday occurrence while simultaneously illustrating that municipal governments—often thought to be corrupt—were actually working well (154). All the while, stories of botched illegal abortions largely remained unspoken.

Women trying to obtain abortions in the United States in the post–World War II years faced increasingly bleak options. Therapeutic abortions became the province of medical boards during this time. These entities sanctioned abortions in particular circumstances and functioned to bolster a defensive medical profession intent on imposing ideological coherence around the issue of abortion, doing so by inventing a notion of pregnancy that constructed the woman as a vessel for an unborn baby (Solinger 1993, 261). Abortion committees became an instrument of directed mistrust toward women who were viewed with suspicion; physicians' newly created judiciary function resulted in professional discourses warning of "scheming" women who could not be trusted when requesting an abortion (251). Solinger (2001) argues that women who tried to pursue legal means of getting an abortion necessarily claimed psychosis, meaning they "had to step into and depend upon the very dangerous, very misogynistic postwar arena of psychiatry in order to construct and justify their request for permission to abort" (43). Women considering abortion faced the procedure and "scare propaganda" that stoked fears of the deadly risks women seeking nonmedical context abortions would face. Naming this fear "terror" and linking it to a new valence of sex-as-unrighteousness and even criminality, Solinger (2001) speculates that much of this angst "must have been stimulated by the sheer degradation of being forced into shameful, shady, criminal activity because one had had shameful sex, because one was willing to mess with what was defined then as female destiny" (40).

Women who were tried in civil court for having sought or having obtained an abortion similarly experienced fear and shame. The abortion trial itself could be a performance of public shaming that involved women watching as their reproductive anatomy was drawn on chalkboards or having to answer probing and explicit, detailed questions about the procedure and their embodied experiences of it. Such trials, then, were spectacles created by men in power to publicly shame women in juridical spaces and before public audiences (Solinger 2007, 156). These various examples demonstrate that those trying to access and receive abortions could potentially find their activity (hyper)surveilled or the reverse—overlooked—based not on concerns of the safety and needs of pregnant women but rather on the political and social preferences of those in power. The indeterminacy of what could happen added to the affective rhetorical ecology of this time, whipping up anxieties of various kinds and by disparate actors all attuned to what was a perceived threat: women's potentially increased reproductive control, their bodily sovereignty, and their ability to rewrite scripts of righteous reproduction.

This brief overview reminds us that the criminalization of abortion was part of larger political, social, professional, and religious agendas—that women's "choice" historically has been tethered to larger patterns of patriarchy and control. By examining two pieces of case law preceding the *Roe* decision, analyzing the *Roe* opinion and dicta, and considering these activities in light of the subsequent Hyde Amendment that curtailed poor women's access to abortion, I disrupt the popular linkage between decriminalization of abortion in 1973 and "women's" agency. I also complicate the narrative of macrochange wherein white feminist movement activity purportedly functioned to "eras[e] the shame and secrecy surrounding abortion" (Reagan 1998, 230). I further use reproductive justice theory to explain how the Hyde Amendment opened new avenues of shaming in this affective rhetorical ecology: namely, shame was effectively transferred onto women who, because they were poor, could not enter the neoliberal market of emerging reproductive opportunities. In addition to centering these vital reproductive justice perspectives on *Roe* and its aftermath, I extend a justice-oriented critique by arguing that the macrochange narrative of choice—especially in the historical narratives related to unwed pregnancy during the twentieth century—rests on a rhetorical construction of agency as essentialized and static—a potentiality that is "a possession or property of an agent" (Miller 2007, 147), a gift bestowed *to* women *by* US Supreme Court justices. When so constructed, agency suggests uncompromised control and choice on the part of the possessor (here, women), obscures the fraught negotiations leading to and the contingent nature of such choice, and deflects attention away from new shaming opportunities that emerge around a choice framework.

Griswold v. Connecticut: *Preserving*
the Sanctity of Marriage

The first Supreme Court decision that linked access to birth control (i.e., the ability to talk to a physician about birth control, much less get a prescription for it) with rights (to privacy) was *Griswold v. Connecticut*, decided in 1965. The case considered the constitutionality of Connecticut's extant birth control law, written in 1879, which stated that preventing conception could result in being fined and/or imprisoned. Doctors and clinics providing birth control information to clients were also held culpable, for the law maintained that anyone aiding in matters of birth control could be prosecuted and punished like a principal offender (Vile 2010, 381).

This criminalization was an application of the so-called Comstock laws of 1873, Connecticut being the only state to still enforce these codes. The laws upheld the notion, cultivated by nineteenth-century anti-vice crusader Anthony Comstock, that sexuality must be publicly managed because sexual desire fomented criminal behavior. According to the logic implied by the law, prohibiting access to contraception was an effective way to manage others' "deviant" sexual behavior or, more specifically, to prevent women and men from having sex without the threat of pregnancy. Ongoing attempts from the 1920s forward to repeal the ban in Connecticut garnered insufficient support in the state senate. Its repeal was especially resisted within the Catholic community (a significant portion of the state's population), which reasoned that more lax birth control laws would create a slippery slope of liberal demands eventually leading to the decriminalization of abortion. Doctors at Catholic hospitals who publicly supported the repeal were terminated under order of the diocese (Hull and Hoffer 2010, 76–77).

The story of how a decision revising the Connecticut law worked its way to the US Supreme Court in 1965 begins in November 1961, when the Planned Parenthood League of Connecticut opened a center in New Haven for the purpose of providing "information, instruction and medical advice to married persons concerning various means of preventing conception" (*Griswold v. State of Connecticut* 1965, 22). The center closed just ten days after it opened on the basis that it was breaking the law by operating as a clinic with the goal of distributing information about birth control (Posner 1992, 206). Estelle Griswold (executive director) and C. Lee Buxton (Yale professor, doctor, and the center's medical director) were both found guilty of violating the state statute. They appealed, eventually sending the case on to the US Supreme Court, which decided that the "law forbidding the use of contraceptive devices deprives married women in Connecticut of their liberty and their privacy, as protected by the Fourth, Fourteenth, and Ninth Amendments" to the US Constitution (*Griswold v. State of Connecticut* 1965, 13).

The *Griswold* decision serves as a critical precursor to the cascade of later rulings that functionally legislate opportunities for fertility management. But the Court's insistence that an exception to the contraception ban could only be made for married couples illustrates the extent to which the ruling's justification relied on marriage as the only sanctioned context for sex. In his opinion, Justice Douglas invokes the sacredness of marriage, lifting the decision above the *kairos* of a mid-1960s sexual revolution and appealing to the *logos* of what he depicts as a timeless and fundamentally human institution: "We deal with a right of privacy older than the Bill of Rights—older than our political parties, older than our school system. Marriage is a coming together for better or for worse, hopefully enduring, and intimate to the degree of being sacred. It is an association that promotes a way of life, not causes; a harmony in living, not political faiths; a bilateral loyalty, not commercial or social projects. Yet it is an association for as noble a purpose as any involved in our prior decisions" (*Griswold v. State of Connecticut* 1965). By advancing the notion of *marriage* as intimacy, the decision situates marriage as the context, rather than individuals as agents, that warrants protection and support.

The appeal to the US Supreme Court amplifies this focus, claiming that a ruling that forbids a married couple to use contraception represents the state having "entered the innermost sanctum of the home." Further, the married couple's right to privacy should be protected because this "home derives its pre-eminence as the seat of family life" and "the integrity of that life is something so fundamental" that it has already served as the basis for protecting a variety of other constitutional rights (14). In short, instead of recognizing that contraception is a concern related to human sexuality and people's bodies and lives, the opinion obfuscates the material realities of sex as a human action with specific, lived consequences. As reproductive justice scholar-activists contend, the ruling established privacy as a "'negative right' to be left alone," which dislodged the right from any contextual factors (e.g., marital status, access, repercussions of medical racism) that would constrain someone from exercising it (Ross and Solinger 2017, 119). This focus also venerates marriage in its abstractions—a covenant of ostensible loyalty, harmony, and endurance.

The ruling also reinforces the perceived immorality of sex outside of marriage. In his concurrence, Justice Goldberg applauds the decision's moderation, asserting that it is a "more discriminately tailored statute" than the earlier ban. The overturned law compromised married couples' privacy because it had reached "far beyond the evil sought to be dealt with"—namely, sex outside of marriage (*Griswold v. State of Connecticut* 1965). The ruling also upholds a particular version of intimacy wherein "intimate acts and choices are either criminal behavior or marital behavior" (Murray 2010). Here "marriage," as an organizing frame that authorizes the privacy ruling, invokes a shared valuation of this sacrosanct institution.

Eisenstadt v. Baird: *A "Mere" Extension of Griswold*

It would be seven more years—with 1972's *Eisenstadt* ruling—before a US Supreme Court ruling deemed individuals rather than the nonhuman unit of marriage worthy of privacy protections, able to inform themselves about contraception and lawfully practice birth control. The criminal law that was struck down with *Eisenstadt* related to contraceptive use but is widely recognized as being a mechanism for expressing disapproval of extramarital sexual activity (Murray 2010). The event that would initiate this change was a public talk about birth control options given to college-age students—a rhetorical performance that would be classified as a crime against chastity, morality, and decency. Just two years after the *Griswold* ruling, Long Island medical student and activist Bill Baird was invited, at the request of students, to Boston University to give a talk on birth control (Kovach 1970). Baird introduced and advocated contraception use as an antidote to global overpopulation, abortion risk, and "the large number of abortions performed on unwed mothers" (*Eisenstadt v. Baird* 1972). Baird was arrested and convicted for exhibiting contraceptives and handing one container to an attendee, which violated the state's birth control laws. Baird's case found its way to the US Supreme Court five years later.

Even though Baird's appeal asserted that the Massachusetts statute violated the Equal Protection Clause of the Fourteenth Amendment by treating married and unmarried persons dissimilarly, the Court's ruling relied on the privacy precedent. Justice Brennan, who authored the opinion, notes that "if the right of privacy means anything, it is the right of the *individual,* married or single, to be free from unwarranted governmental intrusion into matters so fundamentally affecting a person as the decision whether to bear or beget a child" (*Eisenstadt v. Baird* 1972). The privacy statement was not critiqued by any other sitting justices and was subsequently applied to hundreds of federal and state court decisions (Lucas 2003–2004, 43). Although archival records indicate that Justice Brennan agreed to write a short *per curiam* (decision of the Court) instead of a full opinion, not only did Brennan produce a lengthy opinion, he also circulated it on the morning of the *Roe* oral arguments, possibly hoping to influence the outcome of that case (13–14). By extending the *Griswold* privacy ruling to individuals and thus providing a precedent for *Roe, Eisenstadt* bolsters the false notions that the private realm is "vulnerable and virtuous," while the public realm, which includes government and democratic action among citizens, is dangerous and a potential "source of harm or oppression" (Ross and Solinger 2017, 126).

Eisenstadt also rests on the US Supreme Court's inability to uphold Massachusetts' contraception legislation precisely because the legislation was presumably, but not explicitly, based on notions of "appropriate" contraceptive use. Legal scholar Melissa Murray argues that the ruling represents a subtle but powerful court-sanctioned reorientation that breaks open another false binary: intimacy as either sanctioned through marriage or deemed a criminal activity if outside marriage. Because the decision does not explicate affirmative, legal protections for those having extramarital sex even though it does represent a critical shift in the history of unwed pregnancy in the United States, I turn toward the significance of Baird's rhetorical display. This precalculated, rhetorical performance eventually forced the Supreme Court to pinpoint the purpose of a law steeped in an unspecified moralism. Far from just tailoring the extant privacy ruling by a degree, *Eisenstadt* forced the court to parse a law that seemed to covertly regulate sex outside of marriage by denying access to birth control to unmarried individuals. According to one legal scholar, without *Eisenstadt,* "marriage rather than reproductive self-determination would have animated the contemporary view of fundamental rights of privacy and personhood" (Chen 1999, 502–3), a point that while useful, does not consider the limitations of privacy so central to reproductive justice theory.

Baird's presentation was an event coordinated to result in his arrest and call attention to the constraining Massachusetts statute. Details of the event illustrate police officials' vehemence in responding to Baird, despite the eventual confusion over how to properly classify the crime that he committed. According to Bill Baird's memory of the lecture more than twenty years later, approximately 2,000 people attended the event; he was met with "police cars lined up in a row" upon arriving at the lecture hall (Bower 1996). Further, the (scant) discussion of the actions of the ostensibly unwed woman who received a tube of contraceptive foam implies that officials were poised to make an arrest at the first available moment. It seems that Baird was arrested as soon as the woman touched the tube (another object signifying unrighteousness), for there exists no indication that she took any further action or gave any proof of intending to keep much less use it (*Eisenstadt v. Baird* 1972). None of the seven police officers and detectives present bothered to ascertain the marital status of this woman (Lucas 2003–2004, 29). Nevertheless, this oversight ultimately did not prevent Baird's conviction because he, not being a physician, was an unlawful distributor of contraceptives in the state of Massachusetts (*Eisenstadt v. Baird* 1972). Baird had purchased the foam before the lecture from an "18 year old sales clerk, not a pharmacist" at a Boston department store (Bower 1996).

Although Baird made a purchase that the "unmarried" woman ostensibly could have made herself, he faced a sentence of up to five years in jail for having violating the state's "crime against chastity" code. Instead, Baird was incarcerated in a county jail for just over one month (Bower 1996).

By the time Baird's case reached the US Supreme Court, the Justices needed to determine what his crime actually was. The Justices wrangled over the imprecision of the crime, thus Baird's arrest functions as a display of the arbitrary, conflicting, and imprecise legacy of sexual morality legislation in Massachusetts. It also demonstrates how so-called crimes against chastity were considered legitimate enough in the early 1970s to be reaffirmed as such and their violators actively policed, apprehended, and incarcerated. Nevertheless, these illogical laws could not withstand the scrutiny of the US Supreme Court, and subsequently that court's ruling provided a precedent upon which the *Roe* decision would soon be based.

Roe v. Wade *and the Hyde Amendment:*
Agency *"Conferred" and Access Withheld*

As the *Eisenstadt* decision would suggest, the decriminalization of abortion was likely by early 1973, for a precedent had been established for women's right to privacy over issues related to the potential termination of pregnancy. But in 1970, neophyte attorneys Sarah Weddington and Linda Coffee could not sense what the outcome would be for the class-action suit filed by "Jane Roe" on behalf of all US women. Roe was the pseudonym given to Norma McCorvey, an unwed pregnant woman who sought an abortion in Texas, a state that prohibited the procedure in all cases except those that might save a pregnant woman's life. McCorvey did not have the means to travel in order to secure a safe abortion and could not locate an illegal abortionist. Weddington and Coffee, young attorneys eager to challenge Texas's abortion law, identified McCorvey as their ideal plaintiff. The suit was filed under the complaint that the individual rights of Roe, like most women in Texas, were violated because she could not lawfully obtain a safe abortion at the hands of a recognized medical professional (Hull and Hoffer 2010, 115). The Texas court ruled in Roe's favor, but an appeal in December 1971 sent the case to the US Supreme Court. McCorvey, in the meantime, gave birth and surrendered her child for adoption. The *Roe* ruling, stated in Justice Blackmun's opinion, confirmed that a woman's right to privacy encompasses her decision to terminate a pregnancy, thus striking down numerous state abortion prohibitions, and establishing a trimester framework by which states could have increasing power over abortion regulations at later stages of a pregnancy. Although there was a growing national majority that was favoring the decriminalization of abortion, such positions had not yet taken the form of specific state laws (Balkin 2005, 11). Thus, although access to abortions would continue to be a vital issue for many women for years to come, the *Roe* ruling represented a victory for many who favored a legal route to safe abortions.

Although a trope of "choice" permeates varied discussions related to the *Roe* decision, the notion of a pregnant woman's autonomous, decision-making power is not supported by the rhetoric of the Court-issued documents. It is true that in his opinion, Justice Blackmun notes that the right of privacy is "broad enough to encompass a woman's decision whether or not to terminate her pregnancy," adding that the "detriment that the State would impose upon the pregnant woman by denying this choice altogether is apparent" (*Roe v. Wade* 1973). But as rhetorical scholar Katie L. Gibson (2008) notes, the overall tone of the opinion cedes ultimate power to decide on whether to abort to the medical establishment rather than to pregnant women themselves (316). Blackmun writes that the "decision vindicates the right of the physician to administer medical treatment according to *his* professional judgment up to the points where important state interest provide compelling justifications for intervention. Up to those points, the abortion decision in all its aspects is inherently, and primarily, a medical decision, and basic responsibility for it must rest with the physician" (*Roe v. Wade* 1973; emphasis added). It is not necessarily surprising that the opinion would address physicians (here, invoked as male), because, as noted above, in many states the medical profession had recently been forced to follow more strict regulations dictating in what situations an abortion could be legal (Greenhouse 2005, 99). And even though many physicians were increasingly uncomfortable with interpreting vague state laws in order to make decisions about what constituted a "therapeutic," or legally sanctioned, abortion, the medical establishment had long ago vied for power to determine if and in what circumstances women could abort.

Blackmun's opinion functionally erased women from the abortion decision and ceded the ultimate power of "choice" to male doctors. Not only does his wording severely curtail women's agency in relation to abortion, it also suggests that one *rhetorical* (and thus extralegal) purpose of the document might have been to reinforce the power differentials between (male) doctor and (female) patient *at the very moment women* were given "choice." Gibson (2008) argues that by constituting women as patients (and, by extension, pregnancy as an illness), the opinion situates pregnancy and abortion as primarily medical occurrences, functionally silencing the complicated and varied reasons that women consider abortion in the first place. Additionally, the opinion's heavy medical narrative and deference to the medical establishment perpetuates a paternalistic relationship between doctor and patient that "effectively disqualifie[s] the agent status of women, ruling their lives and their gendered meanings impotent in the abortion debate" (323, 327). The relative inattention that the opinion gives to woman's choice has not yet disrupted the strategic white feminist framing despite its many justice-oriented critiques.

A woman's potential agency in *Roe* is further vexed by the malleable term "unwanted child," which appears in the ruling and dicta. Justice Blackmun concludes that the right to privacy "is broad enough to encompass a woman's decision whether or not to terminate her pregnancy," and he goes on to outline several scenarios exemplifying why a woman is better suited than the state to make such a decision about pregnancy. One such example, Blackmun writes, involves "the distress, for all concerned, associated with the unwanted child, and . . . the problem of bringing a child into a family already unable, psychologically and otherwise, to care for it . . . [a factor] the woman and her responsible physician necessarily will consider in consultation." Blackmun situates the idea of the unwanted child within the context of the family, thus suggesting that a lack of "want" extends beyond the mother alone and is contingent on factors, psychological "and otherwise," that might make having (and raising) a child difficult. But by invoking the "responsible physician" from whom the mother can seek counsel, Blackmun's assertion raises the question: for whom is the pregnancy unwanted? Responsibility here implies one's perceived duty to raise a healthy and productive child who will contribute to, not depend upon, the state. This orientation aligns with Michel Foucault's complex notions of *biopower*, which I use here to refer to distributed management of populations within capitalist societies, and the biopolitical, or state-attuned mechanisms for such management. The ecological, sometimes atmospheric effects of such distributed management of bodies can evade detection as they contribute to logics of normalcy and, in the case of this book, righteousness. Likely, the "responsible physician" Blackmun references would help a mother identify herself and her family as "unable" to "care" for the so-called unwanted child—a potential continuation of practices, described in chapter 1, whereby authorities convince women of their assumed incapability to mother.

"Unwanted child" means something entirely different, however, for Justice Byron White, who pens a scathing dissent to the *Roe* ruling. White laments:

> at the heart of the controversy in these cases are those recurring pregnancies that pose no danger whatsoever to the life or health of the mother but are, nevertheless, unwanted for any one or more of a variety of reasons— convenience, family planning, economics, dislike of children, the embarrassment of illegitimacy, etc. The common claim before us is that, for any one of such reasons, or for no reason at all, and without asserting or claiming any threat to life or health, any woman is entitled to an abortion at her request if she is able to find a medical advisor willing to undertake the procedure. (*Roe v. Wade* 1973)

Justice White adds that the Court's decision suggests that the Constitution "values the convenience, whim, or caprice of the putative mother more than the life or potential life of the fetus." For White, fickle women are the mothers of "unwanted" children, and the whims of such mothers devalue life, sometimes "for no reason at all." Women's agency, then, is a primary problem, an unearned and unwarranted affordance that is intensified by the ruling. Clearly, for White, a woman's "life or health" represents the only potential justifications for considering decriminalizing abortion; other reasons are gratuitous and point to a woman's inability to singly (and, it is assumed, appropriately) bear the responsibility (and perhaps the stigma) of her reproductive capacity.

Mention of the "unwanted child" draws attention to want, or desire, as a key component of an abortion decision, even as its various usages complicate an understanding of who does not (or does) want a child and why. This figuration echoes the earlier distrust of women seeking a therapeutic abortion and the public shaming practices of women tried for seeking an illegal abortion; in both cases, women appeal to those in power who bolster their control over women's reproductive lives by sanctioning when and in what cases women are deemed eligible to manage their fertility. This terminology only reinforces public deliberation about the parameters of righteous parenthood while upholding government interests (such as medical authority) instead of truly affirming a woman's positive right to pursue her reproductive desires and determine her wants in relation to her own intimate and unparalleled knowledge of her lived situation.

Additionally, the term *unwanted child*, along with a similar term, *unwanted pregnancy*, had previously figured in reproductive discourses. Specifically, the notion of the unwanted child is one that early birth control advocate and eugenicist Sanger relied upon to differentiate between rich, healthy children (allegedly wanted) and poor, malnourished children (allegedly unwanted)—a figuration that facilitated social control through negative eugenics logics ("Brief for Appellant" 1917). Similarly, "unwanted pregnancy" was one euphemism for out-of-wedlock pregnancy at mid-century, a trope that surely reflected attitudes that unwed mothers should not want to raise an "illegitimate" child. But by the 1960s, the US government began using the term in a wider public health context, invoking it in discussions of disease transmission, overpopulation, and President Lyndon Johnson's War on Poverty (Lord 2010, 122–23). This broader social landscape in which to consider why children might be "unwanted" aligns with an assertion by Celeste Michelle Condit (1990): that women's depiction of abortion rights in popular writing during the years before *Roe* also shifted from discourses of individual preferences (I *want* to obtain an abortion) to the threat of a plethora of undesirable, "unwanted children" leading to social imbalance.

In the wake of *Roe,* abortion rights advocates galvanized around "choice" as a matter of privacy and personal responsibility for the greater (white majority, patriarchal) good, "deliberately moving away from talking about women's rights, sexuality, and abortion" as also relevant to fertility management in an expedient effort to retain broad support among US voters (Fried 2017, 142). As Solinger (2001) explains, in "a country weary of rights claims, choice became *the* way liberal and mainstream feminists could talk about abortion without mentioning the 'A-word.' Many people believed that 'choice'—a term that evoked women shoppers selecting among options in the marketplace—would be an easier sell; it offered 'rights lite,' a package less threatening or disturbing than unadulterated rights" (5; emphasis in original). These observations suggest agency was strongly affiliated with *Roe* in popular imagination, but actually constrained by a pervasive, patriarchal, and white supremacist culture that instead feared women's autonomy and power over their reproductive lives. Fear of the "A-word" is part of the affective rhetorical ecology into which women wrote toward affective realignment, which I explain below. In terms of choice being a marker of real agency, *Roe* effectively demonstrates how agency is "perverse, that is, inherently protean, ambiguous, and open to reversal" (Campbell 2005, 3).

Related to this critique, and critically important to any discussion of *Roe,* is the swift work on the part of lawmakers in the wake of the ruling to limit its affordances through whatever means they had: namely, limiting access to abortion by poor women who rely on Medicaid benefits. By 1977, Congress passed the Hyde Amendment, a perennially renewed piece of legislation (yet to be repealed at the time of this book's publication) originally sponsored by Henry Hyde, a US Representative. Hyde explicitly stated his true desire—to regulate all abortion—and his purposeful use of a Medicaid bill amendment to prevent women from being able to obtain a legal abortion where he had the ability to do so. Before the amendment was passed, US Representative Patsy T. Mink (key architect of Title IX legislation discussed in chapter 2) voiced her concerns with the legislation and urged her colleagues in Congress to recognize it for its lack of justice. Calling the goal of restricting access to abortion "wholly unfair," Mink (1976) argues that the amendment "will not reverse the Supreme Court decision" but will have a "discriminatory effect and ramifications which are bound to be cruel, weighing harshly on those who can ill afford to carry another burden." Mink's plea was not sufficient in preventing passage of Hyde.

Grassroots organizers such as the socialist feminist Committee for Abortion Rights and Against Sterilization Abuse (CARASA) drew from a coalition of activist movements, including those led by Black and Latina women, to oppose Hyde and the 1980 Supreme Court decision *Harris v. McRae* that upheld it. CARASA articulated a fully inclusive approach to reproductive rights and warned that women in capitalistic societies whose privacy rights are protected and who are granted freedoms of choice provided the seeds for enabling differential access. Additionally, CARASA understood that in such a context, resistance to abortion from the New Right could easily leverage the interconnectedness of concerns about "sexuality, work, and family" that could render poor women the target of conservatives (Nelson 2003, 139). These neoconservatives had new fodder as they "promoted a nostalgic vision of the family and women's role within it—a desire to return to the world of June Cleaver and 'Leave It To Beaver,' when female sexuality supposedly remained confined to the boundaries of the nuclear family" (Nelson 2003, 138–39).

Defenses of Hyde have illustrated lawmakers' tendency to frame abortion in a marketplace logic that seeks to normalize the availability of an effectively legalized procedure based on one's ability to pay for it (Solinger 2007, 201–202). As a consumer privilege, abortion-as-choice continues to be an affordance of only some women. Significantly, choice as agency conferred did and does afford new forms of public shaming related to emerging scripts of "good" and "bad" choice-makers. Solinger (2001) argues that as choice became ostensibly rationalized, public discourse increasingly framed "irresponsible" poor mothers as those who should understand their "alleged duty not to choose motherhood" or those who had children but failed to make "good" choices that would allow them to "carry out the traditional civic function of raising future citizens who would be assets in a democratic society" (190–91). Framed as "irresponsibly backward because they were nonusers or ineffective users of birth control" (189), these poor and young women who are often also women of color were explicitly those who, because of the Hyde Amendment, would by the late 1970s experience significant limitations to their reproductive rights and denials of their reproductive safety and dignity.

This reemergence of rhetorical deployments of shame, now directed on non-white women on the basis of their inability to be the capable choice-makers that white and/or middle-class women ostensibly could be—suggests what Sarah Sharma refers to as *differential biopolitics.* Sharma's term reflects an understanding that biopolitics—like agency—is complex, nuanced, affective, and unevenly experienced (Fixmer-Oraiz 2010, 37). Sharma (2009) argues that "the strategizing of invisibility is one way in which biopolitics can be seen as having a differential affective logic" (142); said another way, biopolitics works differently as some people purposefully recede from sight. In relation to the shaming rhetorics that the logics of choice have enabled, invisibility informs this affective rhetorical ecology, but not because of women's strategic effort to not be seen. Rather, women as competent people who are embedded and invested within communities of care and thus able to competently make decisions about their sexual and reproductive lives have been effectively erased—made invisible—within an agency-oriented, differently righteous context. Such a context favors a "dominant poverty narrative" that is "toxic" in its insistence on shaming poor people (O'Hara 2020, 5). Each mention of *Roe* as a decision that gave all women the right to choose (with no mention of its differential applications or its effective reversal in the same decade it was decided) does such erasing.

The depiction of *Roe*'s agential capacity as a culmination of problematic privacy decisions not only selects a partial history of fertility management among women but also enables the myth that the shame of unrighteous reproduction faded because of the ruling. It is more accurate and just to track shame's mutation alongside shifting notions of righteousness at a time of simultaneous rights advancement for women of privilege and a loss of rights for women without such privilege. Further, reproductive justice activists argue that while the impacts of the Hyde Amendment are "wide-ranging and ballooning" (Ross and Solinger 2017, 129), the "Supreme Court has not provided stability or security regarding reproductive law and policy" (127). The myth of agency gained and shame shed relies, in part, on the idealized power of the Supreme Court, its robed justices making decisions that influence the lives of all people living in the United States. Just as trust was placed in the pill as a scientific and medical innovation, I suggest, some of the perceived agency "granted" by *Roe* is enveloped in the rhetoricity of the Supreme Court as an institution of political weight and judicial grandeur. It seems not inconsequential to the prevalence of the *Roe*-as-agency idea that a group of the most powerful men in the nation determined the ruling—and that this agency granted is a formulation of partial freedoms that contribute to persistent fears of the individuals on the Supreme Court being the decisive factor as to the future of abortion in the United States despite the reality that abortion is not presently available to all.

In her discussion of differential biopolitics and contemporary fertility management, Natalie Fixmer-Oraiz (2010) argues that "reducing 'unwanted' pregnancies effectively relocates concern from the *sexual* excess of women to the *reproductive* excess of certain women—namely young, unmarried, and/or low-income women" (39; emphasis in original). My examination demonstrates how sexual and reproductive excess are both emergent fears at a time of technological, legal, and juridical change. Because this change did not result in more affirmative and public uptake of sexual freedom, fertility management, avenues for access, and the trust in women (instead of policing their righteousness as decision makers in a marketplace of increasing choice), it is change that is not sufficiently just. Reproductive justice calls for this public, inclusive commitment—assurances of "*public* support for *private* actions" based on universal human rights instead of adherence to privacy that can be given, rescinded, and/or modified at the behest of governments and others in authority

(Ross and Solinger 2017, 178–80; emphasis in original). In the words of Welch (2004), greater privacy does not result in "having full, publicly articulated and publicly defended reproductive rights and full, publicly assisted access to exercising these rights, since our rights and access currently are very much tied to our economic standing" (21). While such public understanding and support of people's full sexual and reproductive safety and dignity still remains an aspirational goal, turning to sites of microchange located in the public writings of rhetors of the 1970s illuminates key affective struggles among women and suggests ongoing possibilities among wider publics for such justice.

Sites of Microchange: Literacies of Sexual Desire and Reproductive Well-Being

In addition to critiquing the limitations of the pill and *Roe* as macrochange narratives, it is useful to examine sites of microchange—in this case, provocative and subversive writing done by authors of this era who reconceptualized how women might understand and enjoy their sexual bodies. Works by Toni Cade [Bambara] (1970), Erica Jong (1973), Nancy Friday (1973), the Boston Women's Health Book Collective (1973), Katsi Cook (1989), and Barbara Seaman (1969), while not an exhaustive list of rhetors, suggest a range of ways that the sticky rhetorics of persistent shame, fear, and ignorance related to women's bodies were slowly being unlearned and rewritten. The term *microchange* is not meant to diminish the rhetorical force or potential effects of these works; rather, it reflects the pastichelike potentialities of these various texts, which were created for, circulated among, and taken up by various readers and across differing communities. Collectively, these authors' writings extend women's sexual and body-centered literacies—often in ways that acknowledge and/or leverage emotions tied to female sexual and reproducing bodies—thus establishing ways for women to trust themselves and strive toward sovereignty. In this way, such writing performs the rhetorical work of "staking a bodily claim in public," by being "practice[s] of public voicing" similar to what Michaela Frischherz (2015) has examined in more contemporary artistic exhibitions related to women's reproducing bodies and sexual shame (259).

As public expressions working to reorient people from the sticky rhetorics of persistent shame (and fear) about women's bodies, these texts collectively encourage *affective realignment*. I use this term to indicate invited or encouraged shifts in feeling that can be traced through the language and presentation of new ideas about women's embodiment and women's bodies. Such shifts pivot away from negative and oppressive perceptions of how women (and others) "should" feel about women as sexual, reproducing beings to turn toward different associations and more positive feelings of bodily acceptance, awareness, and love. This writing reflects ground-up, collaborative, and woman-centered agency building that people can exercise in community and/or in relation to their communities. Such sites of change should be remembered and honored as being an equally important part of a recent history of righteous reproduction as the technological and legal changes described above.

As I mentioned in chapter 1, Helen Gurley Brown's publication of *Sex and the Single Girl* in 1962 gave voice to two taboo ideas: that women could (and did) enjoy sex and that they could do so outside of the bonds of marriage. Brown's book was both controversial and cosmopolitan. Much of the nation simply was not ready for such frank discussions of (white) women's sexual fulfillment—even by the late 1960s, when the "free love" ideology began to burgeon in coastal cities like San Francisco and New York. But throughout the 1970s, other writers and activists were further encouraging various forms of sexual and body literacies. These various publications punctured silences that long-enveloped women's sexuality and sexual health, replacing epistemologies of ignorance (sites of unconscious unknowing) with new vocabularies and ideas. From imaginative literature to nonfiction publications meant to equip women with specific knowledge, this group of texts enabled women to become more literate about their sexual bodies and sexual selves, thus suggesting, provocatively, that such literacy was healthy and natural rather than deviant and shameful. Such texts also modeled women speaking up and out on behalf of their own sexual well-being and choice; their rhetorical function includes cultivating associations of positivity, knowledge, bodily self-acceptance, and confidence.

Though not a nominally apparent aspect of the burgeoning health literacy movement of the 1970s, affective change is encouraged and warranted through these texts that span imaginative, instructional, and activist genres. Shame is detectable when reading in, around, and through such writing, which is understandable given its stickiness. Such stickiness both reflects shame's ambient presence as a ubiquitous but below-the-radar affect experienced by women and suggests its threatening quality, as Ahmed (2004) theorizes, as a potential site of absorption (90). Intimate knowledge of and comfort in/with women's bodies necessitates eschewing feelings that those sexual and reproducing bodies are sites of disgust that should not be seen, touched, or experienced outside the strictures of righteous reproduction. In other words, if shame's stickiness relates to "what objects do to other objects" (91)—not what they are, then in this case, women's bodies are sites of learned and felt shame because of the threat of the collective power they potentially wield. Said another way, women's uninhibited relationship to their reproducing and sexual bodies was (and is) so threatening to larger structures of gendered, raced, and classed power— changes borne through the imaginary of what liberated reproducing bodies could do—that shame did (and does) stick.

I build my ambient reading of shame by returning to Bartky (1990), who argues that women feel and sense shame *as women* in a manner that is pervasive but that often does not "reach a state of clarity" (95). Explaining how this affect fundamentally infuses gender-based hierarchies, Bartky continues: "Not only does the revelatory character of shame not occur at the level of belief, but the corrosive character of shame and of similar sensings, the undermining effect and the peculiar helplessness women exhibit within their power, lies in part in the very failure of these feelings to attain to the status of belief" (95). People (mostly women as reflected in the survey below) writing to bolster women's positive relationship with and knowledge of their own bodies represent a vital part of the slow rhetorical story of affective realignment away from enduring shame.

As a learned type of gendered experience, shame has recently been theorized in relation to the legacy of *pudeur,* or feminine modesty. Locke (2016) argues that *pudeur,* a French term that in Latin translates to *pudenda* and in German *Scham,* is a historical, cultural, and political philosophy that suggests female appropriateness through sufficient covering (of the body) before others (24). The relationship among these words is revealing. According to poet and literary critic John Hollander (2003), "Germanic languages reached out desperately to cover the nakedness of their bodily terminology with the cloak of Latinity, even to the extent of calling sexual organs *pudenda,* paralleled by the use of *shame* as a noun to designate sexual parts. The Latin *pudenda,* 'that of which one ought to be *or* to feel ashamed or, indeed, ashamed to mention,' was primarily medical usage, and almost always referred to the female genitals" (1064). Indeed, the historical anatomical terminology for "female" external genitalia—pudendum—was only removed from the international dictionary of such terms in 2019, a move that prompted academics to argue over the benefit or triviality of such a change (Draper 2021; Kachlik 2021; Zdilla 2021). *Pudeur* as an orientation across medical, political, and social contexts refers to this concept casting a long shadow. It is "as if the sexual parts of the body, like the sexual impulses of human life itself, shame the rest of the body and the life" or as if some aspects of shame extend shamefulness onto a community or the body politic (1064).

It is not coincidental that shame is addressed in women's writing of this critical moment of body literacy because of the long affective imprint of *pudeur* as well as such writing marking a shift in women's liminality. Shame's relationship to age has been considered by Neil Postman (1994), whose careful reading of ancient texts suggests that shame historically distinguished the young from the mature (9). In other words, insofar as these writings helped women mature into their bodies by way of greater self-knowledge, increased assuredness, and an ability to embrace feelings of worth and desire (sexual and otherwise),

readers were necessarily crossing an epistemological bridge that required acknowledgement of shame's role in this separation.

I consider this project of actively unlearning shame to reflect one type of
ignorance as theorized by philosopher Nancy Tuana. From her examination
of the women's health movement, Tuana (2006) has made the case for dialec-
tically pairing the "complex practices of knowledge production and the variety of factors that account for why something is known" with a simultaneous
examination of "the practices that account for *not* knowing" or the processes
by which knowledge is unlearned (2; emphasis in original). Tuana's capacious
term—epistemologies of ignorance—provides the latitude to explore unknowing across writings from disparate social and cultural locations and writers
uniquely grappling with ways of unknowing that relate to sites of injustice
and/or effects of the long reach of *pudeur*. Shame's presence in various texts of
the 1970s demonstrates the affective epistemological work of these writings as
not only that of "resistance" (7) but of "realignment" of a sticky affect.

Building Political Awareness and
Rhetorical Confidence

In late 1969, writer and activist Toni Cade published "The Pill: Genocide or Liberation?" in *Onyx* magazine. The following year, the same essay was reprinted
in the first publication of a collection edited by Cade (who in that same year
changed her name to Toni Cade Bambara): *The Black Woman: An Anthology.*
Bambara was a Black public figure who contributed to both the women's rights
movement and Black liberation efforts; "The Pill" gives voice to the strained
position of women who navigated between these spaces of resistance. Part of
Cade's work in this short essay is to dismiss the liberatory narrative of the pill,
especially for Black women. She rejects the narrative of instantaneous liberation by asserting that Black women have been "too mobile, too involved with
the larger world outside of the immediate home to be duped into some false
romantic position of *the liberated woman*" (207; emphasis in original). Rejecting outright the universalizing narrative of agency delivered by the pill, Cade
situates the technology within a larger ecology of contentious relations and
a sexual double standard that was evident in the civil rights and Black power
movements. For instance, Cade addresses lore circulated by "women in the
movement" that women affiliated with the Black power movement should not
take the pill "because it encourages whorishness" (206). Cade calls attention to
those women who, when considering pill use, perpetuate shame through an
anti-agency trope: women's control of their own sexual lives is a signal of or a
precursor to their inappropriate (i.e., extant) sexual desire. Cade was initially
"shocked" by this position but adds it to her essay in an effort to help readers
realign away from this logic (206).

Cade continues with her resistance to the easy equation of pill-as-agency-granting for women who consider taking it. She writes, "I would never agree that the pill really liberates women. It only helps. It may liberate her sexually" but "what good is that if in other respects her social role remains the same?" (208). Articulating a vibrant position against agency-as-granted or bestowed upon women by a reproductive technology, Cade asks that her readers further adjust their idea of what the pill can afford. Resisting the pill as a commodified technology for receiving agency, Cade takes a more radical and agency-cultivating approach. "The pill is a way for the woman to be in position to be pulled together," she writes (211). This pulling-together means, for Cade, women developing self-confidence and being able to speak truth to power while cultivating a clearer sense of their own desires as well as how they still exist within systems of sexual oppression and exploitation.

Cade begins her essay with a recollection of a political meeting that offers one model for women taking this critical and structurally attuned approach to resistance. Recalling a "slightly drunk and very hot lady" who, after interrupting the meeting repeatedly was finally asked to speak her mind, Cade explains how this woman leveraged anger and distrust to address the complexity of reproductive agency at this moment. Cade depicts the woman as "righteous and beautiful and accusatory" toward a Black man who chided women to throw away the pill and to use their reproductive capacities to have children for the benefit of Black movement goals (205). Calling out the man on his sexual double standard, the woman asked him "'when's the last time you fed one of them brats you been breeding all over the city, you jive-ass-so-and-so?'" and, with this question, "she tore the place up" (205). With this model, Cade urges readers to see that women have the ability to reconfigure their relationship to systems of power and to predetermined narratives of how they should use their reproductive capacities. Demonstrating that the woman's anger and resistance resonated with her audience while promoting such "righteous and beautiful and accusatory" rhetorical action, Cade provides a model for women to use their voice to navigate the vexed landscape of reproductive politics for women—and especially Black women—in a postpill era.

Wresting Women's Sexual Desire from Gendered Shame

Part of the developing counterculture of the early 1970s was the (primarily and predominantly heteronormative white) women's liberation movement, which found its roots in the organization of small groups of women throughout major cities across the nation in 1967 (Echols 1989, 3; Kline 2010, 14). For some feminists, the goal of liberation necessitated rethinking the relationship that women—and men—had with women's bodies and women's sexuality. At a time when complicity to authority was being interrogated on many fronts, some women critiqued social taboos related to sexuality and sexual bodies. In 1968, for instance, the New York Radical Women published *Notes from the First Year,* edited by Shulamith Firestone (Echols 1989, 60–61). This text included a dialogue of women "rapping," openly and honestly about sex, as well as Anne Koedt's groundbreaking "The Myth of the Vaginal Orgasm." Such pieces spoke out against the notion that women's sexual performance should primarily please men and fueled radical feminists' growing contention that sex was overly influenced by phallic-centered, Freudian theory (Freedman 2002, 263).

Two texts, both published in 1973, put the contentious idea that women did (or should) enjoy sex (and talk about enjoying it) into even wider circulation. Erica Jong's novel, *Fear of Flying,* follows a female protagonist, Isadora Wing, who has a brief affair and gains strength and sexual satisfaction through the experience. The text, a successful popular novel in the United States, can be understood as an imaginative contribution to second-wave consciousness-raising (CR). The CR novel as a second-wave, primarily white feminist genre enables narrative depictions of the process of CR as a "wholly new way of understanding and of making political change" (Hogeland 1998, 23). The book does not only present a fictional world and a protagonist, but it portrays narratively how that main character fundamentally reorients to and resists that world. Jong's text praises the value of anonymous sexual encounters and proposes that women can enjoy and benefit from developing their sexuality outside the realm of marriage and even outside of a recognizable relationship. The disruptive power of the novel comes in part with the *publicness* of Wing's fantasies, an aspect of the text that calls attention to stereotypically masculine fears of unbridled and immodest desires. Jong sets the narrative against the belief that women who expressed their sexual desire in public ways were likely to be seen as impure and unrighteous, as a "contaminating agent for patriarchy, one that explicitly highlights its fundamental lack of control over the female body" (Hood 2016, 160).

Similarly, *My Secret Garden,* Nancy Friday's (1973) collection of real women's sexual fantasies, was an attempt to demonstrate the ubiquity and naturalness of women's sexual thought. Friday's book was an immediate best seller, but its reception was mixed, especially among feminists who did not agree that her belief in "erotic freedom and the shedding of shame" was the necessary conduit to other forms of women's liberation (Bellafante 2007, B13). America's conservative bedrooms were increasingly sites of sexual experimentation and candid desire, as books such as Jong's and Friday's introduced new lexicons of sexual self-expression. A 2013 *New York Times* article on *Fear of Flying* indicates that Jong's work "still has its fervent supporters." Nevertheless, the piece deems the novel a "frank, explicit, chatty account of [Isadora Wing's] quest

for no-strings, satisfying sex" that "electrified and titillated the critical establishment" when it was published (Schillinger). The uneven and ostensibly non-
feminist uptake and remembrances of this work illustrates the discomfort and
labor of shifting from ambient and embedded notions of the proper to new
forms of sexual righteousness that were cultivated by writers inventing new
terms and imaginaries of sexual sovereignty.

Identifying Latent Sexual Shame and Sponsoring Dignity

A central piece of women's reproductive health writing came in the form of
Our Bodies, Ourselves, the health manual produced by a group of mostly white
feminist health advocates who published the first version of the book in 1970.
The authors—the Boston Women's Health Book Collective—helped to make
women's knowledge of their sexual, reproducing bodies a legitimate goal. The
result was a "system disrupting" text (invoking a term theorized by Marika
Seigel, 2014) that reconfigured women's ability to see themselves in relation
to the systems of health around them and not just as patients complicit within
extant systems (DiCaglio and De Hertogh 2019, 565). Such education and advocacy demonstrates how women's writing activities began to overturn long-
held epistemologies of ignorance related to sexuality and reproduction. This
writing also articulates counternarratives meant to reject and revise cultural
logics that expected women to remain unfamiliar with and ashamed of their
own bodies. What would eventually become *Our Bodies, Ourselves* began to
take shape relatively early in the women's liberation movement. In the spring of
1969, one of the first women's liberation conferences was held in Boston at Em-
manuel College, where twelve participants bonded over their feelings of being
dismissed—not listened to or heard—by doctors. Although the group pledged to
continue to meet to develop a list of respectful, informative, local ob-gyns, they
soon realized that a larger project would be more beneficial (Kline 2010, 14–15).
The group continued meeting, researching, and facilitating CR sessions about
topics ranging from menstrual cramps and menopause to orgasm and childbirth (Davis 1983, 21–22). Eventually the group named itself the Boston Wom-
en's Health Course Collective and decided to publish the research and personal
narratives that they had been exchanging. The 193-page, 75-cent version of the
publication was typewritten and mimeographed, featuring hand-drawn images
and thread for binding. In December 1970, the collective published 5,000 copies
of the text, now titled *Women and Their Bodies,* with a local, independent press.
Alternating a collective authorial voice with excerpts of personal narrative
and numerous pictures and diagrams, the text encouraged identification and
exploration. After ten printings, the group revised, expanded, and published
the book as *Our Bodies, Ourselves* with Simon & Schuster in 1973 (Kline 2010,

15–17). Now writing as the Boston Women's Health Book Collective, the group attracted a much wider market of women, significantly building upon its local success. The book had been published continually since that date but in April 2018 the Boston collective announced that it would no longer publish the manual. Having been translated into at least twenty-nine languages, the book has given rise to a host of companion texts and has sold over four million copies (Wells 2010, 1–2).

If novels like *Fear of Flying* and *My Secret Garden* suggested that, by the early 1970s, the sexual revolution could and should be embraced by anyone, *Our Bodies, Ourselves* reassured its early readers that overcoming sexual ignorance and raced notions of sexual shame was a slow, complicated process for women individually and collectively. The authors of the 1973 edition offer that the sexual revolution "has made us feel that we must be able to have sex with impunity, without anxiety, under any conditions and with anyone, or we're uptight freaks," reasoning that such "alienating, inhuman expectations are no less destructive or degrading than the Victorian puritanism we all so proudly rejected" (Boston Women's Health Book Collective 1973, 23).

As an alternative to other texts of the era, *Our Bodies, Ourselves* takes the time and care to articulate the feelings of shame that frequently are yoked with sex. Addressing a paradox of the day, the authors explain, "We are simultaneously bombarded with two conflicting messages: one from our parents, churches and schools—that sex is dirty and therefore we must keep ourselves pure for the one love of our lives; and the other from *Playboy, Newsweek,* etc., almost all women's magazines, and especially television commercials—that we should be free, groovy chicks" (24). The results of these conflicting messages is made explicit in the text, for the authors assert that when men become "sexually aggressive," women "must worry about how to set limits on the sexual encounter" and brace themselves against "this powerful sexuality" (26). More than an early critique of image politics, *Our Bodies, Ourselves* gives voice to the power differential in many heterosexual sexual encounters and explains that an accepted abuse of this power has fostered women's inability to understand their own sexuality. The authors further discuss the tendency toward premature marriage (a result of dominant white culture that values female virginity before marriage), as well as the double standard of men being expected to cultivate their sexual prowess before marriage by sleeping with women who are then deemed "bad girls" (27–28). The collective's willingness to explain these gendered cultural expectations demonstrates its need to bring to light fundamental ideological beliefs of sexual hierarchy in order for women to begin to resituate themselves as more sovereign sexual beings.

Beyond this explication of oppressive cultural logics, *Our Bodies, Ourselves* also provides detailed information on women's anatomy, the process of conception and childbirth, various methods of birth control, and a wide range of topics relating to abortion. Susan Wells (2010) argues that such information represents body education, or one's increasing knowledge of their own embodiment and the need to understand not only one's body, but also that body's social location (108). More than a book meant to shape private acts and private spaces, Wells contends that *Our Bodies, Ourselves* functions as a "grand public telling of secrets" that "opened the public sphere to new issues and new *agents*" (55; emphasis added). Despite having to compose a text that abided by "norms of reticence," the collective succeeded in giving voice to many aspects of women's sexuality that were not otherwise explicitly and candidly addressed in the early 1970s (24).

In 1975, the Boston collective also organized the first National Conference on Women and Health, which was attended by Byllye Avery (2005), who would become "the most recognizable leader" of the 1980s women's health moment among women of color. Avery had helped Floridian women travel north for safe abortions before *Roe* and was the only Black founding member of the Gainesville Women's Health Center in 1974. "Inspired" by the women's health activists she was meeting, she soon joined the board of the National Women's Health Network, an organization that involved members with "radical politics" who "were extremely sensitive to issues of race and class" (Silliman et al. 2004, 64–65). Avery's activism deepened further as she worked coalitionally with the Federation of Feminist Women's Health Centers, a group that "emphasized women's power and knowledge" while advocating for "community control of healthcare" (65).

When Avery noticed that Black women visited the Gainesville Women's Health Center for abortions but not for other reproductive health needs, she collaborated with the center staff to create a model of service that focused on needs of Black and poor women, cultivating an "environment where women could feel comfortable and take control of their own health" and an approach to health care that responded to these women's experiences of "powerlessness" (Avery 2005, 66). Reflecting on the center's goal of offering "body sex" workshops to help women "learn about sexuality," Avery recalls naked workshops in which she and participants "had a lot of fun" but also cultivated dignity: "None of us knew that [our vaginal areas were] so beautiful. And those of us with dark skins, the colors are just beautiful as they go from dark brown to kind of rosy pink to light purple to so on and so." She adds, "We just really sort of gave ourselves permission to learn who we are, to explore who we are to our fullest. And it gave us such a sense of pride" (17). Although I am not suggesting that the Boston collective explicitly prompted Avery's contributions to women's health literacy, I do consider Avery's work to be one important example of literacy cultivation along with the "hundreds" of other books written after *Our Bodies,*

Ourselves, many of which "included differentiated material for women across a spectrum of ages, races, ethnicities, abilities, and sexualities" (Dudley-Shotwell 2020, 8).

Women's health advocates—those in the Boston collective, the National Women's Health Network, and the Federation of Feminist Women's Health Centers among many others—succeeded in drawing attention to systemic problems in the medicalization of women's health and reproduction as well as non-white women's experiences of, in Avery's (2005) language, "liv[ing] in a conspiracy of silence" (66). *Our Bodies, Ourselves* and the community-based uptake of similar self-help and women's health literacies such as that facilitated by Avery persuaded women of the value of emotional reorientation as part of the larger project of cultivating sexual and reproductive self-worth. In *Our Bodies, Ourselves,* this meant being "better friends and better lovers, better *people,* more self-confident, more autonomous, stronger, and more whole" (Boston Women's Health Book Collective 1973, 3; emphasis in original). Women's greater health literacy, after all, needed to be premised on this more fundamental sense of acceptance and dignity of women's bodies, even as affective realignment would not proceed smoothly, quickly, comfortably, or universally across individuals and communities.

Reconfiguring Gendered Relationships to Health

The final examples of affective alignment link two very different versions of women's health activism, both of which sponsored women's awareness of gendered injustices through institutions of modern medicine and both of which encouraged women's rhetorical awareness of their capabilities as knowledgeable actors in their own right. Journalist Barbara Seaman provided an invaluable contribution to the women's health movement through the publication of *The Doctors' Case Against the Pill* in 1969, even though her advocacy had a more complicated relationship with the medical establishment than did that of other white health movement writers such as the Boston Women's Health Book Collective or resistance activists such as Cade. Katsi Cook, whose activism in the later 1970s centered on her Women's Dance Health Program, focused on affirmatively building Indigenous women's capabilities to resist colonial practices of violence and Western assimilation that had "destabilized [these women's] understandings of the meaning of Native womanhood" (Theobald 2019, 166–67). Strategically linking these two activists helps to illuminate how relationships between womanhood, reproduction, and medicine were shifting across white and Native communities in the 1970s.

Seaman began her career as a health columnist for popular women's magazines, but it was her book about the birth control pill that most forcefully called into question acceptance of oral contraceptives in the late 1960s. Compiling a variety of anecdotes and testimonies from both physicians and women who had used the pill, Seaman (1969) demonstrates the lack of consensus about the pill's usefulness and safety. The largest portion of the text provides detailed explanations of the potential complications related to taking oral contraception, including blood clots, stroke, diabetes, cancer, and heart disease, as well as a decrease in the user's sex drive and diminished sexual satisfaction. One chapter serves as an extended case study of a woman who dies from oral contraceptive-related complications. Along with documenting these potential risks, the text outlines why there existed a disparity between the potential harm of the new drug and the limited discussion of these risks with patients. An early chapter, "The Silence That Could Kill You," explains that many physicians lack the time, interest, or moral imperative to fully educate their patients on the potential side effects of the pill. Not satisfied in explaining *why* physicians might avoid informing patients, Seaman also provides a list of characteristics of "conscientious" doctors (17).

Such information not only would have educated Seaman's readers, it also prefigures later work by Kay Weiss (1977), who surveys key forms of education among (male) medical students that perpetuate toxic and shame-cultivating misinformation about women, their reproductive organs, and their relationship to sex. Specifically, Weiss's exposé reveals that medical school literature and pedagogy advance notions such as women being fearful and shame-filled children (even as they give birth), women's feelings of disgust about menstruation based on the vagina's proximity to where the body excretes feces and urine, and a supposed causal relationship between any form of dysmenorrhea with "personality disorders" and/or "neurotic predispositions" (217). These sorts of dispositions and sites of ignorance being folded into medical education suggests the difficulty of Seaman and other activists being heard as relevant and persuasive rhetors, much less the ability for women as patients to reconfigure their own sense of bodily normalcy and rhetorical power in relationship to medical providers.

Physician Hugh J. Davis, practicing gynecologist and John Hopkins professor, provided the introduction to Seaman's (1969) text, thus bolstering Seaman's ethos for some readers despite the text offering extended critique of these very same authority figures. Similarly, by entitling her text *The Doctor's Case Against the Pill,* Seaman elevates the voices of those physicians she interviewed, thus veiling the extent to which the text relies on women's personal experiences to argue against uninformed use of the pill. Despite these constraints, Seaman's voice and vision shaped a book that ultimately questioned the motives and practices of a behemoth, the pharmaceutical industry, earning her the nickname "the Ralph Nader of the pill" (Fox 2008).

Seaman's critique led to Senate hearings on the safety of oral contraceptives in 1970 and an FDA order that risk sheets be included in all packages of birth control pills (Watkins 1973, 4). Although these hearings garnered extensive public attention, women's health advocates were dismayed that no women were asked to testify. And later, the public would learn that one of Seaman's collaborators was Hugh Davis, the inventor of the Dalkon Shield intrauterine device (IUD), a birth control method whose safety was not sufficiently tested in the late 1960s. Davis's IUD led to severe reproductive harm for more than 200,000 women and caused the death of at least eighteen more before the company ceased manufacturing it in 1974 (May 2010, 131–32). Thus, even as influential as Seaman ultimately was in helping women gain access to information about the pill and holding pharmaceutical companies responsible for making a safe product, her story reflects how women's increased agency over their reproductive well-being was complicated by competing interests and situated within an ecology of significant male control.

A very different orientation to reconfiguring women's relationship to their reproductive health comes from Katsi (pronounced Gudji) Cook. Cook (Akwesasne Mohawk), is a significant figure in Indigenous women's health activism whose knowledge as a fourth-generation midwife blended with her interest in the Red Power Movement in the 1970s (Silliman et al. 2004, 125). Cook's long-time work has been to understand Indigenous epistemologies related to womanhood and to address epistemologies of ignorance among Native women due to colonial and biomedical violence. Although those in authority (such as the US government) were responsible for such dehumanizing activity, Cook advocates for Indigenous women taking a more active role in community-controlled health care as a form of sovereignty as key to their reproductive well-being (127–28).

"Women's Dance" was Cook's first piece of published writing, which emerged at the close of the 1970s and reflects lessons she drew from her activism and midwifery training that "could be used to support Native women in a new vision of women's health" (Cook 2005, 67). "Control over production and the reproduction of human beings and all our relations is integral to sovereignty," writes Cook (1989, 85). "Among the Iroquois, the Haudenosaunee, the women 'owned' the gardens, and thereby controlled a major portion of the food supply. Supported by the Clan, the healers, and a community in harmony with the Creation, women had more to do with health than doctors are able to in today's fragmented world" (85). This passage from the text, anthologized in 1989, reflects Cook's interest in reconnecting Indigenous women to their historical and cultural epistemologies of care and sovereignty as well as her ability to configure control as ecological in its situatedness within a wider community and its needs. Comparing her efforts with the Women's Dance Health Program with the work of contemporary white feminists such as the Boston Women's

Health Book Collective, historian Brianna Theobald explains that for Cook, colonization was the fundamental reason that over one-third of Native American women had been sterilized. Cook contends that disparate Indigenous communities need to return to their own ways of knowing less as a matter of possibility and more as a means of survival. For her, "most answers [to this violence] would be found *in* tribal cultures" (Theobald 2019, 167; emphasis added).

Cook hoped to pen a Women's Dance Health Book modeled after *Our Bodies, Ourselves* but written specifically for Indigenous communities. Although the project has never come to fruition, "The Women's Dance" sheds light on the knowledge cultivation and affective realignment of this activist. Educating readers on foundational ideas such as health being "a matter of balance and harmony" for Native peoples (Cook 1989, 81), Cook also reviews sites of lost knowledge about womanhood across Indigenous communities. Offering that in a traditional worldview, "Native American women understood their bodies in terms of the Earth and the Moon," (82), Cook goes on to describe origin stories, puberty rituals, and an illustrative Christian missionary intervention that explains why these traditions were destroyed and must be relearned. The essay further links environmental and human contamination as sites of violence that preview much of Cook's later environmentally oriented maternal justice work.

In making her case for reproductive sovereignty in "The Women's Dance," Cook (1989) also tells the story of being a young girl and catching a glimpse of her grandmother—a source of great traditional, inherited wisdom—sitting on her bed, undressing. She remembers: "Her brown, wrinkled breasts sagged clear down to her waist," a surprising site, as she "had never seen an old woman's breasts before" (88). She continues, "Grandma had felt my child's eyes upon her and she made no effort to hide herself, nor did she show any embarrassment, or an acknowledgement of my presence. At that moment I felt only a tremendous respect for this woman" (88). Replacing body shame with dignity and pride and situating this personal memory within a larger call for Native women to "reclaim our powers on the female side of life," Cook calls for affective and epistemological change among Indigenous women whose traditions encourage self-trust and shame-free power. Like Seaman, she encourages readers to reimagine women's possible relationships with medical authority, while uniquely calling on communal and traditional Native ways of knowing to pursue this possibility.

Throughout the 1970s, a growing number of Americans—especially women—were resisting scripts of easy and equalizing liberation through reproductive advances. They were interested in exploring the idea of sex as being natural and enjoyable and were beginning to reconceptualize sexual and reproductive health as something over which they had a rightful claim to, personally and within their communities of knowledge. The various publications I have cursorily surveyed above suggest that readers' awareness and interests were varied and that creating a discursive space for women's shifting sexual knowledges, imaginaries, and possibilities was a labor-oriented work in progress for rhetors and for readers who contributed to the collective work of change that is less easily remembered than the iconic macrochange explored earlier in this chapter. The gradual shifts in sexual and reproductive epistemologies away from ignorance and shame demonstrated by these texts points to the rhetorical work necessary for affective realignment that could help women envision, experience, feel, and consider their bodies and reproductive lives in new ways that ran counter to long-held notions of sexual shame.

Building from Bartky's work on gendered shame, Sara Cohen Shabot and Keshet Korem (2018) argue that gendered shame "tends to be paralyzing, making women's most intimate embodied selves insecure (384). The pervasiveness of this shame renders the people experiencing it both obedient and disinclined toward social and personal change; the shamed learn to be depoliticized subjects that feel as though they do not have "real agency" (388, 394). If considered a reflection of an "agential momen[t]" these texts, rhetors, and themes, can be considered as "challeng[ing]" contemporary rhetoricians to "think beyond agency as individually and mystically crafted by a volitional subject" (Frischherz 2015, 259) or granted through scientific innovation or judicial decree. Instead, these texts reflect "the conditions that make action possible" (259) and the effort needed to affectively realign away from the sticky rhetorics of enduring, gendered sexual shame.

Threats of Persistent Shame and Misfigured Agency

This chapter set out to complicate the suggestion, advanced by current histories of unwed pregnancy in the United States, that with technological and legislative advances—specifically, the development of the pill and the Supreme Court ruling on *Roe*—the silences related to unwed pregnancy during the 1950s and 1960s fundamentally changed. By exploring these advancements through the lens of a rhetorical feminist historiography of righteous reproduction, I have considered how scientific innovation and a watershed Supreme Court decision helped shape a story about vulnerable unwed and pregnant women and how these public understandings figured responsibility and privacy as loci of control instead of cultivating more communal, inclusive, and affirmative orientations to women's sexual desire and reproductive sovereignty, dignity, and safety.

Ongoing and contemporary efforts to address reproductive concerns about young and vulnerable women further emphasize why attention to what technologically or legally "granted" affordances does not sufficiently address in the complex ecology of material and affective realities. Washington's writing on the history of Black people's relationship to reproductive technologies includes calling attention to the ongoing needs of young Black women whose sexuality continues to be seen as manageable through technological interventions. Washington (2008) admonishes that this approach is short-sighted: "Young girls become pregnant because of a complex set of psychological pressures and risk factors that a pill, a shot, or an implanted capsule cannot address alone. Girls at risk tend to be poor, academically struggling, and naïve about sex and reproduction. They are usually preyed upon and even raped by older men" (209). Discourses that do not attend to complex and troubling realities of women's sexual agency—discourses that rely too heavily on the ongoing affordances of liberation through medical and juridical advancements—fail to help young women today. Dorothy Roberts (2017) has similarly written of the relatively recent use of Norplant to address teen pregnancy (a newer iteration of problematic, intervention-worthy pregnancy that I discuss in the next chapter). Roberts also pleads for readers to understand that the so-called problem of teen pregnancy is "really, in many cases, a problem of sexual abuse, of poverty, of racism, and of inadequate resources for teen mothers and their children" (121). Highlighting the ongoing conflation of technological affordance with sexual knowledge, Roberts rhetorically questions why the promotion of Norplant would be problematic among "poor Black women and teenagers." To answer her own question, Roberts explains that such a strategy erroneously "assumes that Norplant's efficacy at preventing pregnancy means it promotes women's health and reproductive autonomy" (121–22).

Additionally, women who might not have proactively managed their fertility or who, upon becoming pregnant, did not desire to obtain an abortion but still faced carrying a "fatherless" child to term counter the narrative of shame evaporating with the assumed agential gains bestowed to women through sites of power in the 1970s. Just because these women might have had access to abortion does not mean that they would necessarily wish to pursue one, and not pursuing an abortion does not necessarily equate with choosing or being able to raise a child. I have been surprised to come into contact with women who hid an unwed pregnancy and surrendered a child for adoption long after 1973. For example, one woman with whom I spoke surrendered her child in 1982, in part because she wished, as a practicing Catholic, to carry her baby to term. Nevertheless, this woman felt isolated and uncomforted by a family who did not easily overlook the "sin" of her unwed pregnancy. Stories like this one are reminders that agency is always contingent and contextual.

As Amy Koerber's historiographic scholarship on medical approaches to hysteria shows, when women have historically been "grant[ed] a more important role in reproduction," this bestowed agency has resulted in the ongoing "overassigning of agency to females" in situations of unwanted pregnancy and even rape (*From Hysteria* 100). In other words, figurations of agency bestowed through technological, juridical, or other systemic or institutional avenues can be repurposed to oppress women. Even when this reassignment does not happen, granted agency promotes passivity and reinforces individual orientations to agency gains at the expense of more realistic interpretations of the irregular and relational distributions of reproductive autonomy—findings that can be applied to other instances of redistributions of rhetorical agency among those who are marginalized. More pernicious, persistent rhetorics of gendered and sexual shame, when left unexamined, can have a more limiting effect than material barriers to agency. In her study of effects of abortion regulation, Karen Weingarten (2016) argues that shame's tendency to move, transfer, and circulate through bodies "allows it to be a regulating mechanism for controlling populations" (36). Shame's ability to cultivate biopolitical norms of how people relate to their bodies "guarantees that even if abortion is legal or accessible, it will be regulated" and, more significantly, that "shame will regulate those very populations that seek abortion" (36).

Shame lingers and sticks even as publics proclaim that it is disintegrating (for good or ill), even when shame itself functions as the narrative explanation for why the righteousness of reproduction allegedly changed forever. Women's writing influenced the politics of reproductive and sexual health and wellness throughout the 1970s, even if their efforts resulted in sometimes marginal gains against a power-heavy, male-dominated, white medical establishment and entrenched supremacist and colonial social practices. This historiographic revisioning is one avenue toward resisting the myths of agency easily and universally bestowed, problematizing the persistence of rights' relationship to privacy and personal autonomy, and appreciating the complex ways that power functions through language that also, for good or ill, can come to bear on people navigating life as sexual and reproducing beings.

Four

Rhetorical Blame
and Pregnant Teens
in the Late 1970s

'd never thought it could happen to me. . . . What on earth was I going to do now?" These are the thoughts of Terri, the presumably white, unwed and pregnant 16-year-old narrator of a story that appears in the May 1980 issue of *Good Housekeeping*. Writing as a diarist would, Terri describes learning of her pregnancy during a visit to her pediatrician and her resulting fears. "My parents are very strict and old-fashioned. What in the world would they think of me? They'll throw me out! I thought miserably. I was so upset I cried myself to sleep." Subsequently visiting a gynecologist, Terri asks "What about an abortion?" The gynecologist explains that Terri is "too far along," but also chides "Why didn't you see a doctor sooner?" She later describes disclosing her pregnancy to her parents as "more horrible than I'd ever imagined." Her mother and father respond by "shrieking" and demanding to know how Terri could do "this" *to them*. Terri writes that her parents "seemed to assume I'd marry Bill [the father of the baby] and acted shocked when I said I wouldn't." Then they chastise Terri for dismissing the idea of adoption, since her preference "wouldn't be fair to the baby" ("My Problem" 1980, 32).

Pregnant Terri is then cast off by her boyfriend and excluded from parties and gossip with friends. Her story is peppered with memories of "bursting" into tears and feelings of being "utterly rejected." Trying to make sense of how her identity has changed, Terri describes her mixed emotions in light of others' reactions: "Being pregnant proved that I was a woman, not a kid like [my peers] anymore, that I was sexy and desirable. Some of my friends envied my new status and admired me for keeping the baby. Others thought me stupid to get caught" (32). Terri and her classmates orient her situation clumsily among extant and revised tropes related to school-age pregnant women. Terri is refigured from "kid" to "woman," and she perceives that this shift also replaces presexual innocence with sexiness. Her peers judge her as *either* responsible *or* foolish for her behavior and decisions—but always accountable.

Terri's story further yokes responsibility and adulthood, as she emerges as a protagonist poised to choose between embracing righteous responsibility or—already being pregnant—making further irresponsible decisions. Speaking to her nurse about her decision to keep her baby, she insists that the nurse "was calm, friendly, and never sat in judgment," in part because she does not push child surrender. Yet, the nurse quips, perhaps sardonically, that "If you are woman enough to be here, you are woman enough to make your own decisions." She then rehearses to Terri the numerous obstacles that she will face as a single, teenage mother. Terri receives this information with gratitude, beginning her journey toward realizing the righteous responsibility narrative that is the point of the story. Although she is learning about practical matters such as daycare waiting lists and items the baby will need, this advice represents to Terri "the first time anyone had treated me like a responsible person." At a later visit, however, the nurse's warnings tap into Terri's feelings of social isolation. "It's not going to be easy to fit into school life after the baby comes," the nurse cautions. "Oh, some girls manage to study and date. But it usually means they've dumped the baby with Mother and she and Dad are footing the bills. And that's simply being an irresponsible brat" (34).

Apparently having failed at guiding Terri to make the "best" decision on her own, the nurse finally encourages Terri to meet Lisa, the nurse's young sister, who also had a child as an unwed teenager. Lisa's functions as a cautionary tale; being a teen mother is hard; boys will either shower you with attention because they think you are sexually available or avoid you because they think you are trying to find a husband. Lisa admits, however, that recognizing her own seemingly inevitable abusive tendencies as a mother was pivotal, allowing her to realize that she should relinquish her child for adoption. Confessing that "I could barely keep myself from hitting her," which "horrified and frightened me," Lisa explains to Terri that "for my baby's sake, I had to give her up" (36).

The story ends, quite abruptly, with Terri ruminating on her newfound happiness, given her recognition of "how childish and irresponsible" she had been. She admits that Lisa "had put into words a lot of my vague fears," which allowed Terri to decide to relinquish her child. Lisa's counsel allowed Terri to see that she had been "too locked into [her] own viewpoint" and that surrendering her child was "the only responsible thing to do." Her parents now express their respect for her autonomy as a parent, asking her if she is "sure" that she wants to give up her child. Apologizing to her parents for not having taken their needs into consideration earlier, Terri proclaims that she finally realizes that "they *did* love me and want what was best for me and my baby" (36).

I share this extended summary of "My Problem and How I Solved It: I Was Sixteen, Unmarried—and Expecting a Baby" because the narrative compresses the tangle of complications surrounding a post–1970s unwed teen pregnancy into a banal story of self-redemption that illustrates a new righteousness of personal responsibility among young, potentially reproducing women. The short piece, likely penned by a *Good Housekeeping* staff writer given that there is no reference to its provenance, functions dually as an unrighteous pregnancy confessional and as a type of pathography, or a narrative of illness—in this case one that suggests the abusive potential of a young, unmarried, and pregnant woman. Like the pathographies examined by Judy Z. Segal (2005), Terri's story (though fictionalized) humanizes the diseased and ill (60). In sharing Terri's subjective experience, this essay notably brings a young white unmarried mother's voice to readers instead of silencing her and hiding her from sight as was the nearly ubiquitous practice among white communities since the 1950s.

In this unsilencing (of sorts), however, readers encounter an epideictic tale, one that conforms to the ancient rhetorical category of discourse that communicates praise or blame and that traditionally was used as a form of ceremonial high oratory. In studying pathography as an alternative to biomedical forms of communication, Segal (2005) focuses on narrative as contemporary epideictic, referring to it as a culture's "most telling rhetoric, because, in general, we praise people for embodying what we value, and we blame them for embodying what we deplore" (61). Terri's story subjectively recounts her experience and merges medical and moralistic considerations, but instead of analyzing the paradoxes Terri experiences, the narrative maps white and class-based fears of unrighteous reproduction on Terri through her experiences of being shunned, the nurse's admonitory warnings, and Lisa's harrowing tale of self-vilification. The essay concludes with Terri accepting these fears of herself, seeing herself as the "troubled" girl that came to represent young, pregnant women in the late 1970s and subsequent years, despite the differing portrayals of white and non-white girls. Terri fears herself and subsequently chooses relinquishment, thus voluntarily rehabilitating herself by restoring her righteousness—a righteousness that she, as a white woman, can reinstate. Thus, while the narrative celebrates Terri making what is meant to be understood as the correct and responsible decision by relinquishing her child and denying her own motherhood, it also performs a curious epideictic move of enabling praise to covertly deliver blame. In other words, readers are prompted to feel satisfied in a happy ending, but such good feeling comes at the expense of Terri recognizing in herself an irresponsible, even potentially volatile and violent, nature.

Terri's confusion dissipates once she stops courting her own sovereignty and surrenders herself to the paternalized and pathologized role that her parents, the nurse, and her peers see her as occupying, thus making this a tale of double relinquishment. As a pathography not of revirginalization but rehabilitation, the narrative jettisons larger discussions of how the network of adults surrounding Terri might more affirmatively engage "immature" teenagers experiencing unfamiliar sexual drives who may be entering the arena of sexuality and reproduction. The story's parabolic tone implies that the solution to Terri's predicament is a private and prescriptive one: if other girls (or their mothers reading the middle-class, normative *Good Housekeeping*) bear witness to Terri's epiphany, there will be fewer (white) pregnant teens in the first place. The piece also belies the vexed and far-reaching public rhetoric surrounding "teen pregnancy" starting around 1976, when discussions of it as an "epidemic" problem first began to circulate as such. By the 1980s, a national crisis of "babies having babies"[1] fomented growing resentments toward social interventions that directed tax-funded, public monies toward what were thought to be irresponsible, personal failures.

This chapter examines rhetoric about teen pregnancy during four pivotal years leading up to the conservative high tide of the 1980s and focuses on various discourses that index enduring public emotions—shame now apparent as blame and related fears and anxieties—that extend moralizing affect into a moment of emerging, ostensibly rational, and relatively dispassionate social awareness about teenage adversity.[2] With federal protections enabling young, pregnant women and mothers to remain in high schools and colleges, unwed pregnancy among women of all races had become a more visible reality. It could no longer be openly figured as the same shameful public secret threatening racial and class purity standards that upheld notions of whiteness as it had been a decade or more earlier. Yet as Jenna Vinson (2018) has argued, the increasing media representations of teen pregnancy in the 1970s obscured the varied raced and classed experiences of young mothers by visually depicting white teenagers who could be imagined as upwardly mobile through their (relatively) managed fertility.

Young pregnant women's increasing publicness, along with the affordances of contraceptive technologies and the decriminalization of abortion, fomented public anxieties about redeemable and unredeemable teen mothers. The fear of a receding investment in the nuclear family structure—complemented by more incipient fears of all women's potential for greater sexual and reproductive sovereignty—undergirds a shift toward rhetorics of blame leveled at young and differently pathologized women. Because shame did not actually dissolve, it became more publicly toxic, shifting to blame that entwined more openly and more forcefully than before with neoliberal beliefs of meritocracy and responsibility to a free market. Teens like Terri could and *should* follow normative scripts of appropriate (i.e., gendered, sexual, and capitalistic) ways of being. Because these instances of *psogos*, or blame, locate *kakoethos,* or bad character, on pregnant, teen girls—especially those who are unmarried—these women are repeatedly depicted as giving birth to a "cycle of dependency" on the state. Ensuing discourses poised to elicit a generative public response to an "epidemic" of adversity are thwarted, I argue, by their reliance on epideictic rhetorics of blame that insist on teen mothers' deficiencies.

By examining a shift from iterations of private and then more open rhetorics of shame to fully public examples of communicating blame, I engage with an emotion-laden type of discourse that has not garnered sustained attention in ancient or contemporary rhetorical theory (Rountree 2001; Wright 2019). One significant exception is Mark Hlavacik's (2016) work to theorize public blame, or the "spectacular and political" uses of condemnatory rhetoric that circulates and "calls people together to take collective action" (9). Hlavacik argues that any deployment of public blame is necessarily "grounded, explicitly or implicitly, in a set of expectations for ethical action that the accused has presumably violated" (11). Teenage pregnancy discourse exemplifies shame transformed to blame, which allows a rhetorical indexing of blame to render salient such ethical expectations. A public reckoning with purportedly rising numbers of young people becoming pregnant reflects the persistence of a pathologizing sexual double standard in which women are ultimately held responsible for sexual knowledge and consequences even when they are depicted as being psychologically unable to do so (through depictions of adolescent naiveté or being "troubled"). It also demonstrates deepening public shaming practices directed toward poor, non-white, allegedly hyperfertile, or economically nonproductive bodies that I describe in previous chapters. Hlavacik also contends that public blame always "traffics in agency" in ways that warrant scrutiny (10). Young women living in a postpill and post–*Roe* era are variously blamed for inappropriate agency or depicted as unable to assume appropriate agency. The panic resulting from a reported epidemic of teen pregnancy calls forth with urgency a needed public intervention, one that—according to the myth of dissolving shame I have interrogated through this book—does not need to moralize but can instead rely upon reason, scientific detachment, and technocratic solutions.

A pivot to "teenage pregnancy" presents a pressing crisis of public health that infantilizes the teen mother who can be rehabilitated while also casting blame on troubled teens and non-white women for their errant reproduction. This is a complex social moment in which notions of psychological development, depravity, and willful affronts to normative ways of being collide with and foreclose more care-oriented dialogues about girls facing new and ongoing forms of adversity, pointing to the reproductive justice critique of the lack of public uptake of reproductive justice goals and the avenues of support necessary to achieve them. The late 1970s are a time, then, of the fading away of "unwed" pregnancy as an articulated concern and a "redesigning of socialities and intimacies" (Roy and Thompson 2019, 5) for newly figured "teen mothers." In this moment of rhetorical invention, youth are not invited to enjoy "transformative empowerment" as they have since been in the wider reproductive justice movement (Zavella 2020, 140); instead "babies having babies" are over-whelmingly judged and blamed as a new configuration of public shame.

The End of a Decade:
Debating the American Family

Discussions of teen pregnancy-as-epidemic would cast this social problem as a technical quandary for the post–*Roe v. Wade* era, one that could ostensibly be solved by a nation as technologically advanced as the United States. Thus, perfunctorily, such framing seemed to replace older, moralistic concerns of pregnancy outside of marriage at the same time that the so-called crisis war-ranted the scrutiny of pregnant, unwed girls whose bodies were symptomatic of a critical public problem. At this same moment, public health concerns also focused on mental health and alcoholism—conditions that, while connected to biomedical matters, were also understood as representing the more amorphous and socially resonant area of "community health." The nation grappled with a messy crucible of the moralistic, the social, and the medical, and it looked to politicians, spiritual leaders, researchers, and educators for answers and reme-dies.

President Jimmy Carter oversaw a morally infused approach to proactively addressing the "epidemic" that reflected the promise of state-initiated and state-funded, technocratic interventions. Carter assumed the presidency during a period of "stagflation," or high unemployment and high inflation (Flippen 2011, 45). Such economic stress exacerbated the political turmoil of a nation reeling from the Watergate scandal, President Richard Nixon's subsequent resignation, and government-led violence on war protesters such as students at Kent State University in Ohio and Jackson State University in Mississippi. Amid these pressing concerns, angst related to the state of "family" as a US institution was palpable. In fact, "family" served as a central concept of the Carter presidency. Unwilling to eschew the moral implications of "family," Carter nevertheless hoped the nation could agree to using the term more inclusively than before.

A nation devoid of "a strong and stable family life" and its attendant morals, however, was an increasing public worry; a decline in the stability of the "Ameri-can" family was considered the source of all manner of cultural crisis (Flippen 2011, 45). Concern over a frayed sense of family values circulated widely during these years of social, political, and economic difficulty, amplifying worries of the previous decade. Related to these debates were ongoing efforts to ratify the Equal Rights Amendment (ERA), which, if passed, would constitutionally cod-ify rights based on "sex." The ERA galvanized supporters and opponents. Phyllis Schlafly—arguably the most prominent voice of the anti-ERA movement—coalesced support through rhetorical appeals of fear and dystopian predictions. Schlafly claimed that feminists were "'waging a total assault on the family, on marriage, and on children'" (quoted in Spruill 2017, 102–3). This is just one example of how the concept of family was central to gender-related political discourse (and discord) at this time. Reproductive rights and capacities as well as women's roles as connected to their reproductive capabilities were at the nexus of much heated debate.

Given this context, Carter faced a nation much divided and exceedingly fretful; he responded with a values-oriented leadership style (Flippen 2011, 107–9). In his 1977 inaugural address, he pledged to focus on strengthening "the American family," which he described as "the basis of our society." This was no simple or straightforward agenda. A 1978 *Newsweek* article warned of increasing rates of divorce, single parenting, and two-career households. Sites of "institutional interference" by nonparental influences such as television, schools, and peers coupled with the rise of parenting experts further threatened to supplant parents' "self-respect and common sense" (Woodward 1978). Popular discussions of "family" changes (or, as critics would say, disintegration of the family) often and "cavalierly" blamed mothers working outside of the home for a variety of social problems, illuminating the extent to which an acceptable version of "family" depended on gendered logics of "male breadwinning and female homemaking" (Chappell 2010, 161). Pro-family nostalgia, then, was intimately linked to (white) women's economic dependence on (white) men—a dependence that conservatives found acceptable only within marriage.

Amid this nostalgic yearning for stability, so-called illegitimate pregnancy remained a moral hazard to the nation. Capturing a supposed truism of the 1970s, historians Paul Levine and Harry Papasotiriou (2010) argue that "the flowering of the sexual revolution and the withering of the nuclear family created alarming numbers of unmarried mothers" (168). Blaming unwed pregnancy, and more specifically white and non-white unmarried mothers, for the overall "breakdown" of the family resulted in what might have been a largely private issue becoming one of public concern, particularly because of the economic strain poor unwed mothers were assumed to put on taxpayers. *Newsweek* cast unwed pregnancy as a central and very public problem because amid all of the factors contributing to unraveling familial mores, "perhaps the *most* distressing development is the high tide of illegitimacy. Fifteen percent of all births are illegitimate and more than half of all out-of-wedlock babies are born to teen-agers. Illegitimacy is particularly high among blacks: of the 513,000 children who were born to black women in 1976, 50.3 percent were illegitimate. And it is the illegitimate, both black and white, who are most likely to be impoverished, dependent on welfare, deprived of educational opportunities and destined to repeat the cycle with illegitimate children of their own" (Woodward 1978; emphasis added). If "family" was a worthy institution that was faltering, then "illegitimacy," "unwed pregnancy," and "teen pregnancy" were sources of depravity—proof of white, middle-class norms of sanctioned dependency and sexual righteousness having gone awry.

Although Carter hoped that the stability of family could be a bipartisan goal that could foster political unity, the nation was divided on just how *family* should be defined. Evangelical Christians generally held that the only legitimate type was the nuclear family: a married, heterosexual couple with children (biological or adopted). But in this era of dawning (if starkly limited) tolerance of feminism and homosexuality, many liberals envisioned more flexible notions of "families," ones that acknowledged a variety of kinship arrangements, including homosexual partnerships, single-parent homes, and nonmarried co-parenting relationships (Flippen 2011, 103). Conservatives' adherence to a singular definition of family should be understood in relation to the simultaneous focus on an anti-statism sentiment within the New Right, the conservatives who mobilized during the 1960s and 1970s and who gained significant political power with the election of Ronald Reagan in 1980. Such anti-statism exemplified the New Right's "financial and ideological ties to a resurgent corporate-led laissez-faire conservatism" (Chappell 2010, 165). Increased adherence to a free market ideology meant that conservatives targeted welfare programs like Aid to Families with Dependent Children (AFDC), using the pro-family stance to urge that unmarried mothers should not receive federal support. Thus, conservatives held that "without interference by liberal government planners and regulators, the economy would reward those who practiced sexual restraint and marital fidelity with male breadwinner wages" (165).

Given this context, Schwartz (1977) in a *Newsweek* proclamation that "the stigma of having a child out of wedlock has diminished considerably by this time" points to a general belief that the lack of a cultural mandate for hiding white pregnant unwed bodies—that is, the dissipation of the open secret of the shame-based cultural mandate of "going away"—was evidence of shame having largely dissolved. Messages of diminished stigma also explicitly discount remaining sites of shaming, such as notions that poor and often non-white women were birthing cycles of toxic poverty as a form of resentful and willful retaliation for their oppression. As Amy L. Brandzel (2016) theorizes, cultural defensiveness of normativity often configures those experiencing oppression as exhibiting unrighteous "tendencies" (such as sexual lasciviousness), which are then "recoded into rationales for increased state surveillance and state-approved violence" (4). Although this chapter examines a "slower" violence[3] that rests at the nexus of cultural change and, likely, a nevertheless earnest attempt by many to support young women facing adversities (including an unintended pregnancy), Brandzel's point adds dimension to this analysis of what I argue is a moment of inadequate public and state intervention.

For many, *family* encompassed both the promise and peril of a weary nation struggling to redefine itself, and the term, in its varied instantiations, reflected the splintered ways in which Americans were defining themselves by this time. The late 1970s represent a moment where the nation struggled against contrasting, competing versions of itself: was the United States a country invested with a moral imperative of communal responsibility for the good of all, or was it the geopolitical manifestation of a conservative ethic of personal responsibility, accountability, and fundamentalism? These profiles are reductive but instructive, crisscrossed by ideological, political, economic, and religious discourses. It is during this time that the unwed pregnant (and now, allegedly "teenage") body becomes a central figure that catalyzes public attention and debate as to how an epidemic of teenage pregnancy fits into these diverging views of the body politic.

Teen Pregnancy:
A Public Health Problem Is Born

An "epidemic" of teen pregnancy was a late-1970s phenomenon that captured the interest and fear of a nation in cultural flux. Sociologist Frank F. Furstenberg (2010) points to the irony of the panic, noting that the idea of teen pregnancy "rose to a level of public obsession just as rates of teenage childbearing began to plummet in the late 1960s and early 1970s" (1). The incongruity between fact and perception—perception based on apodictic, or presumably irrefutable, proof of a diagnosable problem—points to the manufacture of a newly problematic form of unwed pregnancy. Coverage of the epidemic started as research and then was quickly taken up in the periodic press as well as in communications within relief agencies. Critics—some writing during this time and many more having voiced suspicions in later decades—have insisted that the epidemic was not a crisis at all, but rather a purposeful misreading and misrepresentation of statistical data. Nevertheless, the late 1970s public discussion about teen pregnancy and the ongoing reverberations of the teen mother trope encourages a return to the emergence of the pregnant, teenage girl as source of national concern.

I interrogate the discursive framing shift of the later 1970s while also acknowledging the reality that there was in fact a shift in the demographic of women who received concerted public attention and support for their pregnancies. According to Mary Jane, who worked in a private, secular, residential shelter for unwed mothers in New York City from 1967 to 1975 and who spoke to me about her experiences as a staff member, there was a discernable, quick, and "almost unbelievable" change in the clientele in 1973. Within a few months of the passage of *Roe*, Mary Jane explains, "women" coming to the home were 13- and 14-year-olds, "children" who were pregnant and "scared to death" to even be by themselves at a residential facility, much less to be preparing to give birth. Many of these girls "had no idea how they got pregnant," Mary Jane emphasizes. From the perspective of a staff member, this change was extraordinarily challenging. The language of "babies having babies," which Mary Jane herself uses, helps to explain the disorientation of such a drastic and abrupt transition from working with older, if still often young, women like those I describe in chapter 1. Instead of responding primarily to shame based on righteous reproduction logics, these new clients tended to be experiencing various other hardships such as abuse within the family and substance use. Indeed, it was likely a social service intervention that resulted in them being at the facility. Mary Jane explains that the staff struggled to find a "logical" way to approach and support the new clientele, because as young girls, "they didn't know logic." While Mary Jane understands this shift in residents as correlating with the passage of *Roe,* she also acknowledges that a coordinated turn to supporting these young mothers-to-be was a reflection of social priorities, not a likely change in who was having sex or getting pregnant at any given time. It was not that young people were just now having sex, but rather that with a shift away from practices of "going away," homes and agencies coordinated to identify new young mothers-to-be in need.

Inventing the Teen Mother:
Mediated Constructions of Bad Character

Law and sociology scholar Kristin Luker (1997) argues that the teen mother identity was not so much fact as it was a discursive creation, one that came at a time when "statistics [related to pregnancy] could have been used to tell any one of a number of stories," such as that of increasing rates of abortion among nonteens that Mary Jane's memories confirm (82). Instead, Luker argues that the idea of the pregnant unwed teenager "made a convenient lightning rod for the anxieties and tensions in Americans' lives" at this time (106). A close reading of the rhetorical depictions of teen pregnancy in various publications of the late 1970s illustrates how the issue was framed for general audiences. Teenage pregnancy as epidemic invites readers to envision a necessary and warranted *public response* to a problem that continues to be figured primarily as that of the *teenage girl* who might become or has become pregnant. A range of twenty-one articles devoted to teen pregnancy—addressed to different audiences and published between 1976 and 1980—illustrate the attention the issue garnered. These articles also demonstrate the extent to which a purposely framed, unnuanced, and feared "problem" contributed to shifting rhetorics of public blame. This blame rhetoric further hampered responsive, responsible discussions within larger publics. It also effectuated raced notions of righteous white reproductive capabilities and the perception of non-white women's perpetual unrighteous reproduction as an indication of unreasonable dependency.

As these messages circulated more broadly through media venues, blame directed toward teenage girls amplified. Collectively, these depictions reflect two sites of social blame—a lack of sex education and the putative turmoil of adolescence—but they largely coalesce in gendered blame located in/on pregnant girls themselves. A careful study of blame rhetorics circulating at this time, when considered against the backdrop of changing notions of family, reveals the construction of three iterations of the pregnant teenager, each having her own relationship to righteousness and dependency: the rehabilitatable teen, the troubled teen, and a surfacing version of the welfare queen. I describe each of these figurations below, considering how they animate the "problem" of teenage pregnancy in this purported postshame era.

Though at first blush, the epidemic of teenage pregnancy seemed to encourage a secular, rational, and compassionate intervention in the name of the public good, this tripartite configuration of associations of *kakoethos*—or bad character that undercuts *ethos* (Johnson 2010; E. Miller 2019)—evoked by discussions of "teen pregnancy" as public health crisis suggests a different story. Gendered, classed, and raced scripts of blame locate the pregnant-teen-as-problem and enable earlier expressions of moralistic shame to be reconstituted as a concern over right and wrong versions of female dependency, one with an increasing open investment in preserving free market values. A newly articulated public problem continued to locate the culpability for unwed pregnancy primarily on the unwed pregnant body. When indexed and studied together, these three versions of *kakoethos* suggest that while an overarching framing invited public intervention in the name of public crisis management, a more subtle perpetuation of white purity and class-based morality was enabled through these varied depictions of teenage girls and their differing relationship to rehabilitation, responsibility, and dependency. Taken together, these discourses illustrate how rhetorics of shame mutate into rhetorics of public blame—a move that corrals shame feelings and reconfigures them to agitate the body politic. Such rhetorics stoke the desires and fears of the greater public and ultimately fail to empower women or realistically foster dispositions for considering them as sexual citizens worthy of body knowledge or sexual literacy.

A Problem of Epidemic Proportions: Assessment, Reporting, and Uptake

The "epidemic" trope emerged from Alan Guttmacher Institute's (AGI) 1976 publication of *11 Million Teenagers: What Can be Done About the Epidemic of Adolescent Pregnancies in the United States?* In this 64-page document, AGI, a sister research organization of the Planned Parenthood Federation of America, provides a seemingly scientific overview of teen pregnancy as a newly understandable problem. The report is divided into four sections: a statistics-heavy overview of the state of adolescent pregnancy at the time of publication; a discussion of how a mother's and child's health and wellness are compromised by a teen pregnancy; a sketch of current interventions, including birth control education and the access and availability of abortion; and a vision of what additional interventions might assist in lowering rates of teen pregnancy. An afterward by Daniel Callahan, director of the Institute of Society, Ethics and the Life Sciences, assures that adolescent pregnancy is, indeed, a crisis of "epidemic" proportions (58).[4] The statistical data appear under section headers that function as a primer for contemporary unwed and teen pregnancy concerns, such as "Half of Unmarried Women Have Intercourse by Age 19" (9) and "Teen Mothers Lack Key Skills" (24). Overwhelmingly, the document presents "teen pregnancy" as a troubling issue of and about "teen girls." Of the forty-one total graphs and charts in the document that reflect information about "teens" in relation to "teen pregnancy," thirty-five of these visuals explicitly measure a statistic depicted as relating to females, whereas only six visuals explicitly measure a statistic depicted as implicating males.[5] Although today AGI is a leader in advocating a broad range of issues tied to reproducing people's health, wellness, and rights, the 1976 text enables a valuable glimpse into the recent past and the persuasive and subtle ways that blame tropes can seep into efforts to support girls and others facing adversity in its many forms.

I turn to this "epidemic" frame in an effort to build further on the valuable extant scholarship that analyzes this pivotal document—especially Jenna Vinson's (2018) identification of the report's rhetorical strategies and effects. Quoting from visual theorists Monica J. Casper and Lisa Jean Moore, Vinson argues that the "story told by AGI authorizes experts to speak about and for young women while continuing to focus on women as 'highly visible containers of blame, for societal ills'" (16). I agree with Vinson and further consider the public uptake of this act of rhetorical blaming through explicit arguments and verbal tropes that crystalized sticky, yet heretofore relatively uncorralled, shame-based messages. Subsequent articles on teen pregnancy advance a consistent message that this issue had, in fact, reached epidemic proportions. One uses a dictionary definition of *epidemic* to argue that the claim is not hyperbolic, comparing rates of pregnancy to those of sexually transmitted infections, which are referenced as an undisputed epidemic of their own (Lincoln 1978, 35). An archbishop featured in a 1978 *New York Times* article situated the teen pregnancy epidemic alongside abortion as a key contributor to the nation's "cultural malaise." Not only was the United States experiencing a "surge" in teen pregnancies, according to *US News and World Report,* there was no end in sight to these escalating figures ("Rising Concern" 1978).This uptake buttresses associations between propriety, gender, reproduction, and moral citizen development within a neoliberal context.

By rhetorically constituting the epidemic, the document serves a range of significant persuasive functions. The language of epidemic—aside from being potentially inaccurate—leverages the assumed certainty of medical and scientific language, as Vinson suggests, while obscuring the hortatory undertones that suggest what female bodies should do. Subsequently, the decision to frame teen pregnancy as an epidemic imbued this social "threat" with a sense of urgency that did provoke public notice and response. AGI's report (1976) also perpetuates concern with pregnancy outside of marriage. The document repeatedly references and indexes births "out of wedlock," arguing that these types of teenage births are "especially serious" (18). The document also references increases in sexual activity "from higher income and nonminority groups," citing rates from one "predominantly white" and middle class midwestern city (9). With the invocation of disease and contagion that accompanies the epidemic metaphor, the "social" problem of teenage pregnancy could be reframed as a public health issue that called forth response. Such calls, however, also drew from and advanced racialized and class-based notions of who was already expected to be unrighteous (poor and non-white girls) and whose deviant sexual activity was especially alarming (that of white and more affluent girls).

While I agree with Vinson's (2018) articulation of the teen mother as "preventative subject"—one who "gains recognition only as a lesson or moral for others who should take preventative measures to avoid her fate" and who is "pitied or criticized" (22)—AGI's epidemiological instantiation suggests an unrighteous threat that called forth a sense of rehabilitative potential. Yet by suggesting, while not detailing, preventative public responses such as the need for "realistic sex education," the document continues to ultimately place blame on young women, whose unrighteous pregnancy was apodictic proof of a sexual "problem." In this way, these young women essentially bore the blame for this newly framed social ill. As rehabilitatable subjects, white women especially were in need of a technocratic diagnosis and response in the name of social health. Yet blame remains just that—a communicated message of fault; the conglomeration of blame rhetorics of this time permitted dwelling in the place of emotional responsibility assignment instead of manifesting an actual response based on a perceived health crisis. Paradoxically, the evasiveness of the epideictic/technocratic framing of an epidemic enabled shame rhetorics to morph into a new form that extends a legacy of threatening and unwieldy unrighteous reproduction while simultaneously assuring publics that apodictic reasoning will lead to amoralistic solutions.

News articles reporting on the issue acknowledged a wide range in reported instances of teenage pregnancy (e.g., somewhere between fewer than 1 million and 2 million), but this "curious and unaccountable statistical oversight" did little to call into question the belief that the crisis existed (Slater 1980, 53). A professor of economics featured in a 1978 issue of *USA Today* argued that the epidemic was an invention resulting from erroneous readings of logarithmic graphs, belief in "unpublished tabulations," and the dubious desire for AGI to secure federal monies for the sake of funding abortions (Kasun 1978, 31–33). Nevertheless, questions about the veracity of the reports were scant; it seems as though journalists were persuaded by the sheer bulk of data provided them. Trust may have come from the study's novel and explicit focus on teenagers. Such research was distinct from earlier studies, like those of Alfred Kinsey, whose participants were adults.

Maris A. Vinovskis, deputy staff director to a US House Committee on Population during the late 1970s, witnessed the extent to which the epidemic trope influenced policy discussions during the Carter administration. Alarmed that few questioned the validity of the so-called epidemic, Vinovskis conducted his own assessment of teen pregnancy statistics, finding that the notion of a spike in pregnancy actually ran counter to historical trends. Although Vinovskis (1988) claims that rates of sexual activity among teens increased during the 1970s, the rate at which adolescent girls became pregnant in the years between 1953 and 1978 actually decreased by 44.8 percent, suggesting that the most pressing time to worry about teen pregnancy had already passed (9, 25). Even this statistical information collected about teenage and/or unwed pregnancy before, during, and after the 1970s, including that which Vinovskis provides as an antidote to the misperceptions rampant during the initial years of the teen pregnancy crisis, should be held with skepticism.

The general level of trust in an assessment of an epidemic is less surprising when one considers the apodictic qualities of measurable data used as evidence. In her examination of rhetorical constructions of AIDS, Paula Treichler (1999) argues that when a problem is labeled an *epidemic*, subsequent discourse about the problem is marked by "ideas, metaphors, and images [that] circulate efficiently" (45). Insofar as *epidemic* functions metaphorically to shape audiences' responses to teen pregnancy as a problem, this framing invites an epidemiological assessment of that problem. Specifically, the *11 Million Teenagers* publication implies that the research presented in the document represents a new *scientific* discovery. This sense of an emergent trend—and the AGI's diagnosis of this trend—is bolstered by the brochure's opening excerpt from the "First Interhemispheric Conference on Adolescent Fertility," held in 1976 (7). The brochure explains that "traditionally," adolescent pregnancy had been associated with minority and poor populations, but that "recent *evidence* suggests that teenagers from higher income and nonminority groups are *now beginning* sexual intercourse at earlier ages" (9; emphasis added). Such language decontextualizes adolescent and unwed pregnancy as one aspect of the ongoing history of human sexuality and (re)scripts this issue as a new site of research and professional inquiry particularly as its reach extends to white communities. Although Callahan's afterward briefly explores the broad social implications of a vested and vexed site of moral disagreement, this discussion comes after more than fifty pages of graphs, charts, and other pieces of evidentiary data that suggest adolescent pregnancy is an issue that can be measured, quantified, and systematically dis/covered.

Through this language of pathology, researchers-as-epidemiologists measure and assess a problem that seems to circulate, viruslike, as a legitimate threat to be contained. This approach crystallizes an otherwise diffuse, multifaceted social concern, rendering it diagnosable and treatable. This framing serves, then, as "anti-rhetoric," what Edward Panetta and Marouf Hasian Jr. (1994) describe as discourse that functions to advance a singular, "rational," and "objective" "truth" (58). Such "philosophical or empirical claims to knowledge . . . purport to reveal some truth" and "invite audiences to believe that experts possess a special finding that mandates the acquiescence of other discursive participants," especially because such findings are thought to be "prepared independent of the chaos and politics of ordinary life" (59). The "truth" that AGI's report reveals is a new, scientifically presented, regurgitation of shame rhetorics directed at women. An epidemic orientation demands a locatable source of malady; teenage pregnancy, according to the publication, as this "problem," is often "compounded because births are out-of-wedlock" (7). Through the many charts, graphs, and tables appearing in the document, readers understand that the crisis is measured primarily by considering age and marital status of females; girls' intent is a secondary focus (7–17). Noting that "pertinent information about male adolescent sexual activity is virtually nonexistent" except for "fragmentary survey data," the brochure justifies its decision to "concentrate" on "young women aged 15–19, with emphasis on younger ages where data are available and specific comment is appropriate" (9). The publication portrays sexually active teens as individuals worthy of social protections, education, and support systems; it also underscores their dependency, imploring readers to recognize that "it is the value of *their* [teen girls'] lives, not ours, which is critically at stake" (59; emphasis in original).

The publication's pathologizing technical and medical language also calls for a time-sensitive response while it subverts the social implications of human crises. Treichler (1999) explains that "an epidemic intensifies existing social divisions and codifies cultural stereotypes because there seems to be no time to do otherwise" (45). The urgency of the epidemic of teen pregnancy, thus, contributes to continued insistence that female bodies are the primary site of a teen pregnancy problem—a new version of the sexual double standard of righteous reproduction discussed throughout this book.

Indexing Blame: Lamenting Insufficiencies
and Locating *Kakoethos*

Publics eager to identify sources for this epidemic would encounter varied explanations. In schools where sex education was being implemented, criticisms arose about programs discussing sex in decontextualized ways that rendered them ineffectual and uninteresting to students (Castleman 1977, 551). Nevertheless, a common refrain across many of the articles examined here is "What happened to sex education?" suggesting that the school administrators and teachers were expected to shoulder the responsibility of teaching teens about sex despite the challenges of doing so, among them the gendered, shame-based logics I discuss in earlier chapters. Here I more fully focus on the perception that adolescence, as a developmental phase only beginning to be understood, was part of the teen pregnancy problem. I also examine more nefarious messages that locate the blame of teen pregnancy on young girls.

These figurations of blame take three forms. The rehabilitatable, infantilized teen, notable for her youth and presumably white, was a victim of the folly of adolescence; preventative measures might help her avoid teen pregnancy and young, single parenting and thus repair any potential lapses in developing toward righteous, feminized dependency that would allow her to remain upwardly (socially and economically) mobile. The specter of the troubled teen, however, is also present. This figuration of young womanhood is pitiable, but nevertheless more fear-invoking, for she is figured as being an unlikely candidate for rehabilitation. Overly willful, this teen is unashamed of her current moral poverty and future economic poverty. She is thus a threat to herself and out of time with the typical, if abnormal, understandings of the teenage years. And finally, the malicious willful teen mother, a surfacing version of the welfare queen trope here aligned with teen pregnancy as epidemic, draws upon raced associations between hyperfertility and malevolent, unrighteous, and purposeful or retaliatory dependency. The gendered and raced work of blame as exhibited in these figurations of bad character demonstrate how the intersubjective workings of shame morph into unidirectional configurations of fault that undercut young women's agency, limit their ability to speak back to such deployments of blame, and foreclose avenues for cultivating their reproductive literacy and sexual self-knowledge.

The Pathology of Adolescence

Teen pregnancy, as a perplexing trend, is hardly more confusing than adolescence is, according to a number of the articles reporting on the epidemic. As discussions of the social issue of teen pregnancy become interwoven with discussions of adolescence as a unique developmental stage, depictions of the "crisis" begin to adopt an inflection of age-related disability. Adolescence-as-disability relies upon the idea that the teenage years are not just a transitional phase but represent a time of incomplete identity and non-normalization. The 1970s witnessed an increasing circulation of narratives—such as "After School Special" television programs—that rendered teens as "disabled subjects in need of rehabilitation" because of their status as being "always-already under development." In such narratives, the process of coming-of-age represented nearing adulthood (marked chronologically) and metaphorically overcoming the disabled, non-normative "teenage" state (Elman 2010, 267). Here, my understanding of disability is shaped by Tobin Seibers (2008), who argues that "disability is not a physical or mental defect but a cultural and minority identity. To call disability an identity is to recognize that it is not a biological or natural property but an elastic social category both subject to social control and capable of effecting social change" (4).

Rehabilitation logic participates in the notion that "teenager" is an identity that is not only liminal, but also pathological—precisely because it is marked by nonconforming behavior (Nakkula and Toshalis 2006, 3).[6] This pathology of adolescence, a notion advanced over a decade earlier by developmental psychologist Erik Erikson, emphasizes the universality of the identity crisis as a necessary step from immaturity to maturity (Erikson 1968, 125; Elman 2010, 265). Thus, teenage girls who become pregnant threaten to be arrested in their immature and disabled state. Or as one article suggests, such girls have "already achieved a kind of premature, stillborn adulthood" (Slater 1980, 53).

The teen (as non-normative), then, warrants the concern and/or fear of adults. Further, likening adolescence to disability (however indirectly) demonstrates an ableist orientation that values the "normalcy" (read: nondisabled) of adulthood (Cherney 2011, 10). Such a position is exemplified in Callahan's contribution to *11 Million Teenagers,* in which he urges adults to recognize the "high price" that they are morally obliged to pay to teenagers (Alan Guttmacher Institute 1976). For Callahan, this means that adults should "help [teens] avoid those things we [adults] know will hurt them, help to reduce the impact of those acts (even of folly) which they have already done, help them in a word to make it through the teenage years with as little lasting harm as possible" (58). In an ableist cultural economy, teens are indebted to adults, who have a surplus of wisdom and experience (in terms of both mind and body). This framing of a teen pregnancy problem, then, invites adults to fulfill their social duty in helping to rehabilitate young women—here often depicted as or assumed white—from the threat of veering from the path of righteous (read: married, nuclear-family style) motherhood.

The Rehabilitatable, Infantilized Teen

The most salient depiction of teenage pregnancy at this time is the infantilized figure of the white, young pregnant girl that metonymically stands in for "babies having babies" or "children having children." Articles that invoked this figuration emphasized age and decentered race, thus suggesting a tacit focus on white girls. The rhetorics in these pieces apply two arguments about the gendered quality of blame as evidenced by teen girls who have sex and/or become pregnant: (1) girls are held to a sexual double standard whereby others (particularly male sexual partners) are effectively absolved of responsibility to prevent pregnancy and (2) girls are depicted as being culpable for "ignorance" of their own bodies and reproductive capabilities. These two reasons for blaming young girls work in tandem: girls are too naïve to understand their bodies but they are still held responsible for reproductive consequences that men do not experience.

The sexual double standard circulates through depictions of teenage and unwed pregnancy, albeit in different ways than in earlier years. By the late 1970s, birth control technologies were more advanced and the pill was legally available to unmarried persons because of the *Eisenstadt v. Baird* ruling (discussed in chapter 3). Accessibility of birth control remained a significant obstacle for many women. Nevertheless, lack of knowledge, rather than lack of access, animates teen pregnancy discourse. For example, *11 Million Teenagers* (Alan Guttmacher Institute 1976) includes a discussion entitled "Ignorance, Inaccessibility Main Reasons for Nonuse of Contraception" that focuses on perceptions of "teenagers," such as the assumption that "time of month, age, or infrequency of intercourse" make contraception "unnecessary." The section concludes by stating, "Contrary to some conventional wisdom on the subject, only one in 15 [girls] said that they did not use contraception because they were trying to have a baby, and only one in 11 indicated that they wouldn't mind getting pregnant" (30). Thus, the "conventional wisdom" about girls who get pregnant outside of marriage—that they are purposefully trying to do so and using (or not using) contraception strategically to that end—is noted as erroneous but left unexplored.

Additionally, this description advances the notion that girls might not want to get pregnant, but it retains a focus on them—a gendered application of blame that stokes fears of the consequences of unmanaged female fertility. The document fails to address boys' responsibility in obtaining and using contraception, much less the gendered power differentials perpetuated by notions of "proper" female comportment. At best, girls are expected to guard their own fertility in order to civilize boys, who are, as a *Seventeen* article explains, under "a great deal of pressure" to "perform sexually to supposedly prove their manhood." Thus, "girls can help show them that manhood can and does mean a lot of other things" (Wax 1978, 173). At worst, girls are expected to transcend overpowering sexual encounters.

One presumptive expert[7] featured in *Reader's Digest* claims that "many girls think it's 'all right' to have sex if they have been seduced or overwhelmed," and thus "they fail to prepare themselves." According to this reasoning, any "failure" that results in teen pregnancy rests solely with girls (Naismith 1977, 152). Such a response not only assumes that girls have access to methods of "preparation," but also—and more problematically—ignores the gendered asymmetry of "seduction" and obscures a reference to rape with the euphemism "overwhelmed." These writings, then, engage in a form of victim-blaming that seeks to identify intentionality and locates it on those reproducing people who, if and when they become pregnant, make visible an unrighteous behavior.

Some of the depictions of young, pregnant girls emphasize what was referenced in the *Nation* as "appalling ignorance" about "the basic facts of their reproductive systems" (Cherlin 1978, 729). Such blame locates deficiencies related to body knowledge and contraceptive technologies on the female, not on technologies, their dissemination, or a dearth of ways to cultivate sexual and reproductive literacies. A 1978 *McCall's* article discusses girls' misinformation about risks related to the pill and IUDs, additionally noting that "only" 41 percent of girls surveyed could correctly identify, according to the rhythm method of contraception, the time when they were least likely to conceive ("The Teen Pregnancy Epidemic" 1978, 45). *Newsweek* suggests that the "plague" of teen pregnancy stems from teens' "confusion about what constitutes a sexual act" (Schwartz 1977). Such statements measure women's knowledge as an accepted way of addressing this "plague" even though, as I argued earlier, teens are repeatedly rendered irresponsible and immature; indeed, discussions of the need for contraceptive technologies to evolve to better address the current "crisis" were mostly absent from this discourse. An article from *Ebony*, a publication that claims to provide an "authoritative perspective on the Black American community," provides a more balanced critique: "behind the national statistics testifying to the proliferating number of adolescents giving births, a perplexing question remains unanswered: Why do teen-agers *permit themselves* to become pregnant? Why, in this age of easily available birth control devices, do young Black girls and boys let their sexual activity lead to conception?" (Slater 1980, 56; emphasis added). Conveying bewilderment, this passage blames girls but nonetheless encourages readers to assign fault to any and all young people who, according to this logic, should have full awareness, literacy, and control over their reproducing bodies.

By focusing on ignorance, and primarily that of girls, these discussions pay no attention to hard-won and recent advances in women's knowledge about their bodies and reproductive technologies—epistemological inroads that resulted from the women's health movement described in chapter 3. Given that the movement gained momentum only a few years earlier, teen girls' ignorance about sex and their bodies is unsurprising and could have been framed as a reasonable consequence of a shifting and shame-prone orientation toward women's sexual identities and the affordances of emerging technologies and legal rights. Nevertheless, the fear and misunderstanding exhibited by young, sexually active girls is depicted as an insufficiency of the group, rather than one implication of contraceptive technologies' complex history. Worse, this misunderstanding is configured as a shameful marker of female ignorance. It is the doctor's impatience with Terri's ignorance that prompts him to ask her why she hadn't come to see him earlier in her pregnancy in the story that opens this chapter; Terri's ignorance creates an aperture for this question, which delivers shame and blame, not information or assurance. Teen pregnancy should simply be prevented and when girls who lack literacy fail at prevention, they should be rehabilitated into righteous modes of feminized dependency.

Penning a *Reader's Digest* editorial, Eunice Kennedy Shriver (1977) also invokes a sense of adult responsibility for helping teens—in part because of the pervasive notion that their identity is pathological. Shriver responds to another columnist who writes that "short of locking the entire teen-age population in their rooms, the only thing adults can do is help them avoid the most permanent and disastrous of consequences—pregnancy" (Shriver 1977, 153). This depiction of adolescence as an abnormal and dangerous time that must be endured likewise advances the notion that adults must "help" teens brave the illness of this liminal age and suggests that teens' danger lies in their sexual capacities and proclivities. Shriver finds these comments "shocking" and "demeaning" in part because they imply that teens "are without values (or that what sexual values they do hold are nothing more than raw pleasure principles)" (Shriver 1977, 153). Yet Shriver's perspective is unique among those I have located. Attending to the teenage years as a ubiquitous, if confounding, phase of development ultimately blames young women—and especially the nonminority teens reputedly prompting this intervention—in a manner that renders the illness of adolescence temporary. (White) babies having (white) babies leverages innocence and racial purity to enable the eventual restoration of "good" white girls who manage their reproduction for the (economic) good of wider publics.

The "Troubled" Teen Girl

Other depictions of the teenage pregnancy problem figure young girls as more disturbing and volatile actors in a contemporary milieu of community health concerns. Such girls are either willfully disobedient, so psychologically fragile that they have a problematic lack of control, or a mixture of both oversubscribed and insufficient agency. For instance, an article in a 1977 issue of *Newsweek* describes pregnant teenage girls as being "a different breed from their cliché counterparts of a generation ago: more sexually experienced at a younger age, better informed about birth control but not necessarily more concerned, and far less scandalized by pregnancy" (Schwartz 1977, 54). In depictions such as this one, girls as a "breed" *willfully* become pregnant for dubious reasons. Additionally, teen girls (as immature/undeveloped adults) are characterized as being—actual or inevitable—abusive or neglectful mothers.

Comparing these more disturbing iterations of teenage pregnant girls to those that primarily focus on the folly of youth suggests a fear of girls who could not be effectively rehabilitated because of a willful independence or psychological abnormality. The rhetorical quality of such figurations is especially apparent when one considers that they echo arguments about the psychological illness of unwed mothers as expressed in the 1950s and 1960s (Solinger 2000) as well as one name for unwed mothers—*incurables*—that circulated in earlier decades. These depictions weave through wider discussions of teen pregnancy and thereby indirectly hold the "troubled girls" against a normative standard of "proper" girlhood that values sexual ignorance and (a)sexual innocence. Girls who deviate from this norm, as suggested in these articles, are also to blame for the epidemic. Locating blame on these more nefarious young women aids in differentiating between those girls who are essentially threatening and those girls who must be protected from (and rehabilitated past) their adolescent deficiencies.

Examples of the troubled girl type include those young women who "choose" to become pregnant because they are purposefully seeking motherhood. *Seventeen* magazine reports that birth control availability and education is of little concern to these teens, who "deliberately" get pregnant ("The Teen Pregnancy Problem" 1980). Another article cites a Los Angeles-based head obstetrician who argues that girls purposefully get pregnant in an effort to produce "a doll" that can serve as a "love object" or to retaliate against their parents (Slater 1980, 56). The *Nation* opines: "The teen years are frightening. The world looks huge, cruel, and incomprehensible; the economy is in trouble and teens feel it directly in chronic unemployment or dead-end jobs. Becoming a parent is much easier and more fulfilling than finding work—any work, let alone meaningful, satisfying work. For many teens, a child gives them personal dignity, something to do with their lives, someone to love and someone to hold power over in a world where they feel powerless" (Castleman 1977, 551). Whether these diagnoses suggest a professional psychological assessment or lay observations about the reasons teen girls get pregnant, whether they suggest pity, empathy, or disdain, they all ultimately participate in epideictic rhetorics of blame that hold girls culpable for willful disobedience.

Not only do these depictions warn readers of girls' childish self-interest (instead of embracing an ethic of care), some profiles emphasize the girls' violent proclivities. One "expert" argues that with "rare exception," young people are ill suited to parent and that this can lead to "outbursts of violence with the infants as the victim" (Marks 1979, 30). In another article, the medical director of the New York Foundling Hospital, who is touted as being "a widely recognized expert in the field of child abuse," claims that young unwed mothers often "become saturated with a sense of desperation, alienation and anger" that "leads them" to abuse their child ("The Teenage Pregnancy Epidemic" 1978, 48). Again, one is reminded of Terri's story and Lisa's confession of nearly abusing her child, which prompts Terri to recognize her own propensity for violence. Such depictions caricature teen mothers as uniformly grotesque and mentally unstable, an act of othering as pathology that can be diagnosed in/on the body.

Also notable in light of portrayals of willful and troubled teen girls are changes that took place in residential care provided for teen mothers in this era of allegedly shame-free sexuality among (also allegedly) younger and younger people. In 1976, the Florence Crittenton Association, (a mission that provided residential maternity care since the late 1800s) merged with the Child Welfare League of America, an organization with a wider scope in addressing youth welfare needs. The merger aligned with another variant of the teenage pregnancy problem of the late 1970s: the "troubled" teenage girl who exhibited a range of behaviors including drug use, criminality, and running away from home ("Florence Crittenton Mission" 2019). A new Crittenton Center in Kansas City, Missouri built in 1977 focused on what it considered was the unmet need of girls whose deep psychological impairments made them a threat to themselves, their communities, and to the unborn children they might have.

In a promotional document for the cutting-edge facility, the Kansas City center contextualized its evolving mission. "Today, Crittenton continues its tradition of rescuing young girls: not from 'white slavery' as in the 1890's; not from the social stigma of unwed motherhood; but from *themselves.* Because of intolerable frustrations and unmet emotional needs, our girls are lonely, confused, and often angry or bitter." Describing the young women who come to this facility, the document notes that "only one in ten [girls seeking help from Crittenton] comes from a natural mother/natural father family unit" and that "most" have "failed and no one wants them" ("Imagine Being" 1977). The cover of the document reads "imagine being in a world of nowhere" and features an abstracted and graphic rendition of a photo appearing inside the booklet of a girl with her arms and head on her knees (fig. 5). This poignant text depicts teenage pregnancy as an isolated girl in need in an effort to raise funds for a capital campaign. This depiction amplifies fears of willful deviance and suggests that some girls are a threat to others and themselves, operating outside of

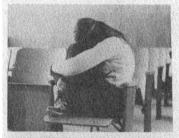

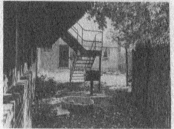

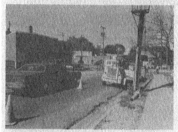

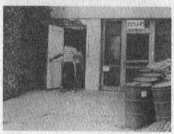

Our Girls

"I wanted to change, but I didn't know how . . . each time I went back to the same old thing because I didn't know what to replace it with . . ."

"I learned to make a lot of decisions that, had I not been here, I wouldn't have had a chance to make. I wouldn't have even known that I had the choice."

"Some of the rooms don't even have windows."

"I might have been dead by now . . . I was really into drugs . . . I didn't care about anybody."

"For recreation, we go up on the roof and watch the cars go by."

Our Staff

" . . . not having the ability to just go and sit under a tree, to climb a tree . . . to sit in the grass and look at the clouds and be in touch with that sort of thing."

"Once they get in touch with their feelings and can look at their pain and look at their sadness and loneliness that's underneath the anger, then they can start controlling themselves and building skills."

"The main advantage of the new facility will be having the physical structure that we need to do our job."

Figure 5. Images representing "Our Girls" from a Kansas City, Missouri, Florence Crittenton publication, ca. 1977. The quotations likely describe the experiences of the nine out of ten girls who did not "com[e] from a natural mother/natural father family unit at the time of admission" and who may have spent time in at least one "institution." Social Welfare History Archives, Child Welfare League of America Records, series 3, series 3.1, box 106, folder FCD Executive Roundtable Meetings, 1977, University of Minnesota Libraries.

the typical timeline of the already pathological phase of development known as the teenage years. Like the Alan Guttmacher Institute, the Florence Crittenton Association (a now reconfigured and renamed justice-oriented organization still in existence to which I return in my concluding chapter) aimed to help girls in need, even as the rhetorical framing of such help reflects logics, associations, and values of this moment in the recent past. Interventions (including residential care to remove them from other children—an echo of earlier spatial rhetorics of hiding and erasure) assumed a different intensity; such teen mothers posed a legitimate threat to themselves because of their very existence. The specter of these deviant girls reminds that their continued contact with others is a fearful proposition and, more generally, that the threat of unmanaged teenage sexuality could have far-ranging consequences.

Appearing within a larger narrative of teen pregnancy-as-epidemic, these constructions identify a tragic, yet simultaneously willful or psychologically broken, figure whose presence calls forth unspecified, fearsome effects of nonprevention. Undisciplined by the nuclear family, left to explore their natural proclivities, these girls display a most base and pitiable form of girlhood—but one that is to be taken seriously even if their troubles exceed a more generic and public intervention. Troubled girls thus serve a rhetorical function within the epideictic frame, reminding of the cost of nonprevention and the perils of white adolescence uncontrolled.

The Malicious Teen Mother

Blame rhetorics take on an especially significant role in these public discourses when the economic costs of teen pregnancy is highlighted because of the ways that blame articulates to racialized tropes of economic productivity and dependency. Dependency, a theme at the crux of the concern around "babies having babies," assumes a double register at this point. For young white women, who were the visible representations of the epidemic as Vinson (2018) has argued, dependency is amplified by the move toward infantilization I describe above. This depiction of dependency racializes the concern over problematic, young white women who might have babies while unmarried. These young women represent non(economically) productive bodies and improper forms of (gendered) social dependency. Nevertheless, they are essentially rendered *malevolently errant*—a public health threat to be intervened upon and rectified. This is an important distinction in part because it makes salient the moral and raced underpinnings of the epidemic.

According to Vinovskis (1988), by the late 1970s, "the real problem of adolescent pregnancy for most Americans [was] not the number of pregnant teenagers, but the increasing proportion of out-of-wedlock births" among this group (28). Specifically, between 1960 and 1977, the rate of births to unwed mothers aged 15 to 19 years increased by 64 percent. Additionally—and significantly—this increase aligned with a perceived demographic shift: unwed teen mothers were much more likely to be non-white than white. By 1983, argues Vinovskis, four out of ten white teens who gave birth were unmarried, whereas "almost nine out of ten births to nonwhite teenagers were out-of-wedlock" (28–29). Of the 34 of pictures of females in the *11 Million Teenagers* brochure, thirty appear to be white[8] and four appear to be non-white, demonstrating that as a status, unwed/teen mother was functionally white-washed within the uptake of the epidemic narrative.[9]

Discourses of teenage pregnancy, then, should be interpreted alongside circulating figurations of Black motherhood at the time. A 1977 Philadelphia, Pennsylvania, Florence Crittenton publication emphasizes a post–1960s shift in providing residential services; once the agency helped (white) "girls who had nowhere to go," but now it was assisting "girls" who needed help for "other reasons" and because they "came from homes where there were multiple problems" (*There Is Time to Think*, 1977). The accompanying illustration replicates a desire for anonymity but communicates a non-white clientele (Fig 6). However, more pernicious depictions of Black unwed mothers as an unassailable source of poverty that were allegedly sapping the economic resources of the nation haunt more widely circulating, public discussions of teen pregnancy as a problem necessitating public intervention.

A prevailing image of Black unwed motherhood—coalesced in the widely circulating stereotype of the "welfare queen"—lingers and reemerges in the context of the epidemic as a threatening and racialized variation on the teenage mother theme. The "welfare queen" identity is what political scientist Ange Marie Hancock (2004), drawing on other scholars including Patricia Hill Collins, refers to as "the indigent version of the Black matriarch controlling image" and "a dominant mother responsible for the moral degeneracy of the United States" (56). Hancock further details the caricature: "She is judged at all levels to be shirking her duty to carry her part of the load as a citizen. She usurps the taxpayer's money, produces children who will do the same, and emasculates the titular head of her household, the Black male. In the language of the national family, she avoids contributing her fair share to the national well-being, either as a 'bearer of American values' or as a contributor to the US political economy" (60). This identity was specifically public—that is, it is one that circulated in news depictions and in discussions of poverty and economic policy. The depiction is what Hancock refers to as Daniel Moynihan's hegemonic "sociological interpretation of the Black poverty problem" (59). The image influenced perceptions of poverty and race among political liberals and conservatives, and it shaped various communities' attitudes about single and poor Black mothers.

RECOGNIZING THE NEEDS OF THE GIRLS

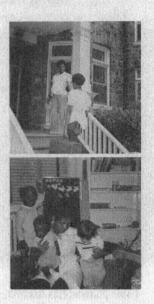

In the late 1960's, Cultural and Social changes lessened the demand for residential care for unwed mothers. However, reassessment of community needs identified an **UNMET NEED.**
...RESIDENTIAL TREATMENT for adolescent pregnant girls who had **NOWHERE** to go.

We found there were girls who still needed a residential setting — but for **OTHER REASONS**. They came from homes where there were multiple problems: marital-economic-overcrowding and misunderstandings. They came from foster homes (65% of our girls) and some from more than one foster placement.

They were uprooted many times.

They needed a **PLACE** and **TIME** to **THINK** and work out their personal problems, feelings, family relationships and **PLAN** next steps.

To meet **THEIR NEEDS**, agency programs had to be reevaluated and modified.

Figure 6. Image representing a new clientele of "girls" from a Philadelphia Florence Crittenton publication, ca. 1977. Florence Crittenton Collection, box 23, folder 12, University of Minnesota Libraries Meetings, University of Minnesota Libraries.

While age functioned as a primary and foregrounded measure of problematic pregnancy in the late 1970s, the specifically racialized threat of the "welfare queen" mentality taking root among a greater number of young women—even white women—haunts this discourse of teen pregnancy. Despite claims that the shame of unwed pregnancy had dissipated, many of these articles reference teen mothers' marital status and link unwed pregnancy with a mother and child's reliance on welfare. Thus, along with other supposed abnormalities, teen mothers were frequently associated with unproductivity and dependency (in relation to society). For example, although such discussions frequently reference the unlikelihood that teen moms will graduate from high school, these references typically frame the dropout problem as one that contributes to a lack of job skills or general productivity. One article simply states, "teenage mothers are less likely to be working and more likely to be on welfare than mothers who first give birth in their 20s" (Lincoln 1978, 36), while another purports that "teen mothers tend to drop out of high school and to survive on welfare," adding that "they rarely develop marketable job skills" (Castleman

1977, 550). These references lament a lack of self-sufficiency and subsequently highlight teen mothers' failure to fulfill a social obligation rather than critiquing social systems that force them to choose between being a mother and being a student.

By insisting that teen pregnancy frequently leads to welfare dependency, depicters of the epidemic also frame teen pregnancy as a problem that represents a quantifiable economic "burden." According to the *Reader's Digest,* "A teen-ager's out-of-wedlock baby generally affects everyone who pays an income tax or sales tax." This is because "society spends an estimated $2,250 each year to support a mother and one child on welfare—plus additional amounts for medical care, social-service workers, and aid to any other dependent children the mother may have" (Naismith 1977, 151). In another piece, a Cornell University psychologist laments that "these people [unwed mothers] are going to put a growing burden on our society, not only to sustain them but to repair the social and economic damage they do" ("Rising Concern" 1978, 59). Girls who have babies out-of-wedlock are girls who begin a "drift toward dependency" that ends up "cost[ing] taxpayers about 6 billion dollars a year in welfare payments" (59). If the moral shame related to unwed pregnancy had at all subsided by the late 1970s, these statements demonstrate how a resentment-fueled notion of dependency took its place.

Aligning unwed pregnancy with dependency did not reflect "mere" economic "realities"; instead, this dependency trope invoked a host of negative associations, all of which cast teen mothers as a deviation from and a detriment to the normative, able, and productive body. Nancy Fraser and Linda Gordon (1997) trace a genealogy of the concept of dependency in US history and argue that the notion of dependency is so shrouded in shame that any adult who is not perceived to be an able worker "shoulders a heavier burden of self-justification" in our independence-obsessed culture (131–35). Additionally, *dependency* functions as a feminized, racialized, ableist term that has historically shifted back and forth between identifying an economic state and insinuating a "moral/psychological" deficiency (131–34). Building upon the notion of a "poverty-shame nexus," Elaine Chase and Grace Bantebya-Kyomuhendo (2015) argue that poverty is not an absolute but rather a rhetorically understood phenomenon; that is, poverty is "understood not solely in terms of whether there is enough food to eat or clothes to wear, but whether people have the resources to adequately function within a society, to play the roles of mother, father, community member, and citizen." Suggesting poverty as a frequently moralized and/or experienced abject state across cultures, they add that "within the vacuum created" by a lack of resources "the fecundity for shame and shaming is likely to emerge" (2). Despite this tendency, shaming remains a rhetorical choice when it is directed (in this case as blame) and used to delineate a class of people based on how their reproductive unrighteousness suggests their ability to reproduce poverty as debasement.

Significantly, these depictions of teen pregnancy also appear after an alarming shift in depictions of US poverty that took place in the mid-to-late 1960s. While the demographic facts of poverty did not change during the decade, greater media attention to poverty during the latter half of the 1960s involved a racialized—that is, racist—pattern of depicting poverty as Black. In fact, news media coverage that included pictures of the poor rose from 27 percent of images depicting Black people in 1964 to 49 percent in 1965, 53 percent in 1966, and 72 percent in 1967 (Gilens 2003, 110). Simultaneously, such media depictions often used images of Black persons to illustrate stories addressing themes such as welfare abuse and nonproductivity (113). While these depictions focused on both men and women, the consolidation of concern about welfare dependency on the Black mothering body cannot be denied. Adjacent to a national concern over an "epidemic" of teenage pregnancy was the conjuring of the vilified, pregnant, or mothering and unmarried Black "welfare queen."

At this time of racialized depictions of poverty and unrighteous dependency, Ronald Reagan was honing a narrative that would further direct blame to Black mothers. When campaigning for governor of California in 1970, Reagan promised to work toward eliminating welfare fraud, and by 1976 he started sharing an anecdote about a Chicago "welfare queen." The story of this woman who gamed the welfare system in order to collect more benefits than she was due invoked racist sentiments and exploited a politics of resentment. The "welfare queen" trope, although offering no explicitly racial language, was often associated with an African American woman, Linda Taylor, who was tried for welfare fraud in 1977 (Cannon 2000, 457). Popular among many audiences, the trope became exceedingly familiar and, according to Hancock (2004), media depictions of the "welfare queen" consistently link her with insufficient industriousness and hyperfertility—long-held associations that were present at the time of slavery. These depictions affirm Fraser and Gordon's (1997) assertion that the poor, single mother has long been "enshrined as the quintessential 'welfare dependent'" (134) as well as their claim that African American women receiving public funds were thought to be "pathologically independent with respect to men and pathologically dependent with respect to government" (138). As Patricia Hill Collins (2000) argues, the African American "welfare mother" who is "typically portrayed as an unwed mother" is a "woman alone" and thus her vilification "reinforces the dominant gender ideology positing that a woman's true worth and financial security should occur through heterosexual marriage" (79).

The invocation of dependency in articles depicting pregnant, unwed, teenage girls operates within a double register. Specifically, dependency here evokes what Fraser and Gordon (1997) call the "bad, relief sense of dependency" but covertly promotes a "good, household sense of dependency" (134). In other words, dependency on welfare is maligned because it is thought to be a marker of individual deficiency rather than a necessity based on a variety of socioeconomic factors (131). But hyperattention to teen pregnancy intimates that these girls deviated away from a "proper" dependency on a male breadwinner, such as a father or a husband.

Pregnant Teens Enduring Blame

As mentioned above, women's increasing autonomy was thought by many to be contributing to a transformation of the American family, and for conservatives, especially, this change was unwelcome and fear producing. The late 1970s experienced a backlash against New Deal and "Great Society" programs—programs whose spirit of extending public support to those in need replaced older methods of granting welfare entitlements only to women who passed "morals tests" proving that they were not sexually promiscuous (Gordon 1994, 298–301). This "economic and ideological shift" from a "postwar consensus" marked a public commitment to move away from resource redistribution and "social safety nets for all" and to move toward tolerance of "speculative finance, deregulation, and the fetishizing of the so-called free market" (Roy and Thompson 2019, 4). Public relief opportunities of the earlier twentieth century based on sanctioned public needs allowed single mothers in later decades to rightfully apply for welfare benefits. To some, however, this equal affordance connoted the public sanctioning of unrighteous behavior—that these mothers were being rewarded for having nontraditional families. By the late 1970s, some presumed a crisis of authority in relation to patriarchal norms that upheld the value of female dependency on men and the supposed universality of the nuclear family. At the same time, neoliberalism was gaining traction, particularly given Carter's deregulation of the economy. As the US economy seemingly sputtered, various unwed pregnant bodies became symbols of unrighteous dependency and the "willful" or "ignorant" state of adolescence. Thus, "dependency," as the term circulates in these articles, is "overdetermined" insofar as it collapses these "multiple" and "contradictory" meanings into one word (Fraser and Gordon 1997, 123). Just as the idea of chronic welfare dependency amplifies the fears related to teen pregnancy, so does the figuration of girls as hyperdependent children evacuate the discussion of overt references to race while inviting a "benevolent" response on behalf of innocent, infantilized girls facing adversity. This response depends on teen girls' sexuality being arrested and their figurative reversion to a state of immaturity. As one child psychologist reports in *Newsweek,* "We must accept responsibility not only for the little girl's child, but for the child in the little girl" ("Pregnant Teens" 1977).

As teen pregnancy became an increasingly public issue, unrighteous management of fertility as a burden on the public good prompted a public desire for diagnosis of the problem of teen pregnancy and, more specifically, a diagnosis of the girls who were ultimately to blame for it. With the idea of the epidemic firmly taking hold in the public's mind, the Carter administration decided that an intervention was needed on behalf of the American family, the children of teen mothers, the mothers themselves, and—not least of all—the taxpayers who would finance the "cycles of dependency" that teen pregnancy created.

A Public Response: The AHSPPCA and
Rhetorical Inadequacy

In June 1978, Joseph Califano stood before a US Senate committee, assuring his audience that "adolescent pregnancy is one of the most complex, persistent, and poignant problems facing our society today" (Adolescent Health Services [Senate] 1978, 23). Califano headed the Department of Health, Education and Welfare (HEW)—a precursor to the Department of Health and Human Services and Department of Education, both of which would be created the following year. HEW had crafted a new bill—the Adolescent Health, Services, and Pregnancy Prevention and Care Act (AHSPPCA) of 1978—that sought to direct federal monies toward the problem of teen pregnancy, Califano being its most ardent champion. With a proposed $60 million appropriation in a time of austerity in many other areas of government spending (the equivalent of more than $245 million dollars in 2022), the bill was meant to prevent initial and repeat teenage pregnancies, to provide care to pregnant teens, and "to help adolescents become productive independent contributors to family and community life" (Adolescent Pregnancy 1978, 2).

The AHSPPCA generated two sets of hearings in the House of Representatives and one hearing before the Senate Committee on Human Relations. Backed by the Kennedy Foundation, the AHSPPCA gathered support from a broad coalition of groups all committed to addressing teen pregnancy (Mittelstadt 1997, 330). The legislation proposed a wide range of potential services, including health, educational, vocational, and social services initiatives; as such, it was similar to other HEW-backed projects that had the capacity to burrow into the fabric of communities to address politically volatile public health and welfare issues.

The AHSPPCA represents the Carter administration's most interventionist response to the supposed epidemic of teen pregnancy. Examination of congressional testimony about the bill, as well as the legislation itself, demonstrates how this intervention did indeed tap into issues that were simultaneously social, economic, medical, and racial. It made good on Carter's declaration that teen pregnancy was a top priority on his domestic agenda (Mittelstadt 1997,

329). As such, the bill—and the more than 1,000 pages of congressional testimony about it—presented an opportunity to shape a conversation about teen pregnancy that would not only result in the AHSPPCA passing through Congress but also its cultivating a mindful, robust response to the alleged epidemic. Although the AHSPPCA succeeded in obtaining the full appropriation for fiscal year 1979, funding was not renewed. By 1981, the Adolescent Family Life Act (commonly referred to as the Chastity Act) became the new legislation for teen pregnancy intervention and ushered in an era dedicated to replacing sex education with abstinence-only education, halving the budget for this effort in the process (Mittelstadt 1997, 331; Valenti 2009, 111). At the end of the 1970s, then, in the wake of legal and technological gains in women's reproductive autonomy, an intervention on behalf of young women can be understood as a retrenchment in distrust, fear, and women's sexual shame that has, in some ways, endured since that time.

The AHSPPCA's reliance on a rehabilitative framework promotes the productive (able) body as the benchmark toward which adolescents should strive and situates the pregnant, teenage body as a threatening deviation from this norm. Its use of rehabilitative discourse perpetuates a myth: that the problem of unwed pregnancy can and should be fixed and that such fixing should be directed at the non-normative, pregnant, teen. The rhetorics of blame present in varied popular depictions of teen pregnancy are also present in the AHSPPCA, and Califano and other key speakers rely heavily on blame when framing the bill and the congressional hearings. This epideictic display of blame collapses the varied invocations of the teen mother while delimiting the deliberative potential of the hearings, constraining an opportunity for dialogue by remaining fixated on the current epidemic instead of envisioning a realistic response to this complicated social "problem."

Califano's testimony before the Senate Committee on Human Relations presents the initial, and perhaps most fully articulated, expression of HEW's proposal to respond to teen pregnancy. He opens with the significance of the bill: "Teenage pregnancy—the entry into parenthood of individuals who barely are beyond childhood themselves—is one of the most serious and complex social problems facing our Nation today. For most of us, the birth of a child is an occasion of great joy and hope, and investment in the future, a consecration of life. But for hundreds of thousands of teenagers, particularly the majority who are unmarried, the birth of a child can usher in a dismal future of unemployment, poverty, family breakdown, emotional stress, dependency on public agencies, and health problems for mother and for child" (Adolescent Health Services [Senate] 1978, 18). This presentation of teen pregnancy as a dire social problem relies on some of the same language of failure, decline, and the drift toward dependency that circulated in popular discourses described above. It also affirms that marital status, along with age, contributes to this "most serious and complex" social problem.

Califano's depiction explicitly locates this downward spiral on young, unwed mothers, suggesting that their pregnancy is a harbinger of perpetual failure and overreliance on the state. The language of the bill itself marshals existing anxieties about unwed pregnancy and reminds that nearly one million adolescents became pregnant in 1975. Further, the AHSPPCA claims that adolescent pregnancy is "often" responsible for "severe adverse health, social, and economic consequences" including "a higher percentage of pregnancy and childbirth complications; a higher incidence of low birth weight babies; a higher frequency of developmental disabilities; higher infant mortality and morbidity; a decreased likelihood of completing schooling; a greater likelihood that adolescent marriage will end in divorce; and higher risks of unemployment and welfare dependency" (Adolescent Health Services [House] 1978, 3). Here, the adolescent body is a monstrosity because it is both sexually mature but not mature enough to birth healthy, able-bodied babies. This liminal, pseudoproductive status of pregnant teen girls is also anxiety-producing because of its reliance on public funds. Repeatedly, adolescent pregnancy is tagged as being a risk factor for repeat pregnancies, which are threatening because they extend the dependency horizon and allude to indefinite cycles of poverty. According to this logic, unwed pregnant girls not only deprive the nuclear family unit, but they are inadequate proto-citizens as well. In short, they fail themselves, their children, their families, and the greater society who now has to bear a burden for "their" reproductive actions. While this depiction does not explicitly invoke race, in it one can register echoes of the pregnant teenagers in the three keys discussed above. Such statements, delivered at the end of the decade, might invoke varied and overlapping associations: the fear of increased teenage sexuality among nonminority teens, the specter of the "troubled" and potentially criminal young woman, and a revulsion toward the increasingly raced and feminized depiction of poor women as the source of economically oppressive, unapologetic, and therefore malevolent dependency.

Teen Pregnancy: A Fixable Problem

In explaining the "dimensions of the teenage pregnancy problem in America," Califano points to the decline in the age of puberty, but he only reports this decline in relation to girls. "The average age of puberty in the United States today is 12.8 years for girls, but about 13 percent [reach] puberty at age 11 or younger," the Secretary warns, adding that this means that "some children reach puberty by the fifth grade" (Adolescent Health Services [Senate] 1978, 19). By using the average age of female menstruation to measure the "dimension" of teen pregnancy, Califano positions the adolescent female body at the center of this crisis.

Because teen pregnancy is repeatedly localized onto the pregnant girl's body (even though Califano and others periodically note its larger social reach), solving this problem can and does assume a rehabilitative tenor. Oriented to resolution rather than accommodation or empowerment, this approach decontextualizes the various forces contributing to teen pregnancy and demands girls' self-regulation while espousing a "comprehensive" solution. Thus, the testimony is framed as an opportunity to move efficiently toward outcomes. For instance, Senator Edward Kennedy, the bill's sponsor, explains to the Senate committee that "we will hear why even when family planning services are available to teenagers, some utilize these services and others do not. We will hear why so many young girls, who are still children themselves, become pregnant a second, third, or fourth time, and we will hear how comprehensive adolescent pregnancy care centers have been successful at preventing these tragic repeat pregnancies" (Adolescent Health Services [Senate] 1978, 42). Kennedy suggests that explanations and solutions are already available and that the testimony only need move, linearly, toward the enactment of the AHSPPCA. This rehabilitative frame relies on the presumed simplicity of a problem-solution orientation that ignores systemic injustices to assure that the disability of teen pregnancy can be overcome.

Such assuredness notwithstanding, the AHSPPCA and its backers fail to deliver on this rehabilitative framing. Moreover, testimony before the House Committee on Education and Labor calls attention to the limitations of this rehabilitation framing and of the testimony to learn from those with valuable first-hand knowledge. Chris Mooney, a director of a program for young mothers and a former "young student mother myself," proposes that abortion be addressed more fully in the bill, since abortion functions as a viable option for many pregnant teens who find their situation "a difficult road to travel" (Adolescent Pregnancy 1978, 57–58). Mooney also reminds listeners that the freedom of choice should include the option of keeping a child, and she urges committee members to consider how "by making remaining pregnant such a difficult option, we are abridging this freedom for many young women" (58). Critiquing the bill's emphasis on providing contraceptives to teens, a solution that she notes is not supported by research, Mooney advocates further study with the hope that new "approaches" (not solutions) might be developed (60). Perhaps most tellingly, Mooney ends her testimony with her "greatest concern," which is that the problem is being approached "overzealously—as if we were 'stamping out' an infectious disease." Reframing the "problem" entirely, Mooney offers that "pregnancy is a normal outcome of normal sexual activity. Teens need to see their procreative abilities as a wonderful, powerful gift which must be intelligently used in the context of their goals in life" (60). Mooney thus illuminates how the threat of "teen pregnancy" hinges on the construction of unnatural, exceptional bodies. Borrowing Rosemarie Garland-Thomson's (2011) definition of disability as "a pervasive cultural system that stigmatizes certain kinds of bodily variations" (17), it is fair to say that Mooney also suggests that pregnant, teen bodies are rendered disabled by this framing. Mooney's statement confronts legislators with a call for breaking a blame-driven frame, working past the apodictic obsession with rates of pregnancy to collectively invent opportunities for women's empowerment, self-knowledge, and sexual sovereignty.

Also shedding doubt on the supposed problem-solving capabilities of the AHSPPCA is Karen Mulhauser, then-executive director of the National Abortion Rights Action League (NARAL). Mulhauser contends that the bill and Califano's testimony both are "exceedingly ambiguous" about the AHSPPCA's priorities, which is particularly problematic given that the requested allocation remains "very small when put against the general purposes of the bill" (Adolescent Pregnancy 1978, 117). In addition to critiquing the frequently referenced yet undefined term *comprehensive services*, Mulhauser also makes clear that the bill wholly fails to address "the involvement or responsibility of the adolescent male" in relation to this "dire" problem (118).

Attending to the internal inconsistencies of the bill and its presentation to Congress makes salient one important way in which the rhetoric of the AHSPPCA failed to take advantage of an opportunity to reframe and meaningfully respond to teen pregnancy. The AHSPPCA hinges on rhetorical depictions of constrained teen bodies despite its reliance on the idea of self-actualizing rehabilitation. Mulhauser, for example, notes how the bill limits the range of possibilities for the teenage mother, a limitation that aligns with the deterministic language mentioned in the articles discussed above. Specifically, Mulhauser argues that according to Califano, "90 percent of the life script for a teenage mother [is] already written for her" (Adolescent Pregnancy 1978, 119). Laying bare the AHSPPCA's "bitterly ironic" logic, Mulhauser explains that the proposed intervention is based on a linkage between teen pregnancy and "pervasive social problems" but completely eschews a discussion of "abortion or access to a full range of alternatives counseling" (Adolescent Health Services [House] 1978, 119). Mulhauser's observation exposes how pregnant, teen bodies are the focus of this intervention, but seem to function as part of a goal that places constraints on what their pregnancy can and should mean. In Mulhauser's opinion, "To be provided with full information about all options available so that the pregnant teenager can make her own choice is the only fair way to deal with a situation which, as even the Secretary has testified, can be totally devastating to her life and future" (Adolescent Pregnancy 1978, 119).

The irony that Mulhauser makes salient suggests that the AHSPPCA actually attempts to preserve a compulsory notion of "normal" sexuality within marriage. The bill assumes a rehabilitative approach to teen pregnancy because, as an expression of compulsory righteous reproduction, it cannot normalize a spectrum of iterations of pregnancy that includes the unwed teen mother. Robert McRuer (2006) argues that this type of compulsion uses the "appearance of choice" to veil a "system in which there actually is no choice" (7)—an observation that aligns with reproductive justice calls for reproductive human rights for all people, including young people. Such a justice-oriented approach contends that sexual desires of young people are natural (if not universal) and thus not alarming; additionally, young people can be entrusted to participate in shaping a sense of who they wish to be as (potentially) reproducing people. Thus, while the AHSPPCA seems to advocate a plan for working with teen mothers as they assess their options during and after their pregnancy, it actually constrains these options. In so doing, the bill indirectly promotes the "propriety" of the traditional nuclear family and fails to heed the calls of young parents and their advocates.

Dependency and the Threat of Unproductive, Reproducing Bodies

Similar to what appears in other descriptions of teen and unwed pregnancy, the refrain that teenage mothers are destined to be dependent on welfare is written into the AHSPPCA and peppered throughout the House and Senate testimonies. Kennedy, for example, contends that teenage pregnancy "imposes a terrible burden on the girl, as well as a social burden on society" because "for over half these girls, the birth of a child begins a cycle of dependency upon public welfare" (Adolescent Health Services [Senate] 1978, 42). The senator adds that the bill makes sense "from a dollars-and-cents point of view," because it is meant to keep "young people away from the dependency on the community in terms of welfare or other social services" and will "permi[t] them to gain employment or to continue employment" (41).

Even after taking this position of advocacy, Kennedy asks Califano to make a stronger case for the funding request, hinting at the issue's intersection with race- and class-based prejudices. Kennedy's is a lone voice in gesturing toward the volatile intersection of race, class, entitlement, and sexual propriety, despite its articulation of presumably wide-held public judgment: "I think what has to be on the minds of an awful lot of Americans, is how can we . . . think about a new program that is targeted on people who are generally the poorest people in our society, and in the lower socioeconomic range of our system. This, of course, does happen to others in the higher incomes but generally what we are talking about are children of welfare mothers. The attitude that is abroad, at least in some parts of the country, is that this particular group of young teenagers—perhaps some people in middle America question their moral values or standards" (Adolescent Health Services [Senate] 1978, 44). In response,

Califano insists that, above all else, this is an economic matter, and diverting money to a solution "will save this country not simply untold human suffering, but tremendous amounts of money over time" (44). Such discursive dancing points to the persistence of moralizing that, when subverted to concern with the economic order, can be understood as reconfiguring righteous reproduction.

The portability of a body metaphor (an analogy that shuttles from the physical body to the body politic) and its ability to marshal support for legislation addressing social liability is illustrated as Califano continues: Teenage pregnancy "tremendously scars the individual girls. It scars her in human terms, obviously, but in economic terms, she becomes less productive for our society; she has much more difficulty getting employment; there is a much higher unemployment rate among girls who have babies, and they earn much less over the course of their lives. So I think this investment . . . will pay enormous dividends for the American people" (Adolescent Health Services [Senate] 1978, 45). Figuring the maternal body as the site of production and reproduction (for the sake of economic productivity) reduces the woman to her womb and upholds a patriarchal valuation of woman's laboring, reproductive capacity—a view of reproducing bodies as vessels of labor power that should produce more labor power. Thus, an overarching goal of the AHSPPCA is not to better learn about, understand, or respond to unwed pregnancy comprehensively, in its various, localized iterations, but to supplant welfare dependent bodies with productive ones.

Even as an initiative backed by the Carter administration, the AHSPPCA's deep commitments to neoliberal tenets of deregulation, free markets, and the dismantling of social programs rhetorically exhibits an allegiance to ableist and patriarchal orientations. Such a position might have appealed to a variety of members of Congress—those who wanted to see rates of teen pregnancy decline and neoconservatives, in particular, who were advocating antistatism and the market's ability to be a moralizing agent. This perspective also helps to explain Eunice Kennedy Shriver's insistence that she and other AHSPPCA supporters are "not just trying to get [girls] back to school, and we will. We are not just trying to get them into jobs, and we will. We are trying to encourage them to respect themselves and to understand their obligations to society" (Adolescent Health Services [Senate] 1978, 115). This discourse points to how such an intervention itself bolsters larger trends like "the feminization of the US labor force and the decline of social services triggered by neoliberal economic policies"—a concern investigated by Anne Teresa Demo (2015) as she theorizes the rhetorical relationships between motherhood, consumerism, and capitalism (6).

By limiting discussions of the AHSPPCA to the epideictic, the bill's proponents cordoned off opportunities for moving beyond blame, identifying with pregnant teenage girls, and revisioning ways to address teen pregnancy (even when witnesses, like Mooney, provided generative, counterapproaches that reconceptualized the situation). Epideictic rhetoric refers to oratory of display that focuses on the present and amplifies "the virtue or vice" of a current situation (Rountree 2001, 296). Epideictic typically addresses the orthodoxies and heresies of a culture and, in so doing, articulates the boundaries between "us" and "them." Rather than making a reasoned argument or introducing audiences to unfamiliar information, epideictic reinforces what an audience already believes about itself (Sullivan 1991, 231–33).

Thus, as a discourse of "conformity," epideictic, by definition, deepens a sense of identification among hearers (by praising those like them and/or blaming those unlike them) and dissuades dissent (Murphy 1992, 72; Sheard 1996, 766). Because of these characteristics, epideictic is considered a particularly fitting style "for addressing private and public dis-ease" and discomfort with the status quo (Sheard 1996, 766), but an inappropriate or ineffectual type of rhetoric for moving audiences to make decisions (Hauser 1999, 15). Epideictic's attention to *doxa,* or popular beliefs, ensures that it references abstract, transcendent ideas of a community but not necessarily factual claims grounded in material realities that can be skeptically and rigorously addressed (Sheard 1996, 774). Although the AHSPPCA seemed to frame teen pregnancy as an economic, technological, and educational issue (rather than a moralistic one), its failure to ultimately move past blame is illustrated in a telling and distasteful statement published in the *Nation:* "When it comes to reducing the teen pregnancy rate, [HEW] appears to be as sophisticated as a 13-year-old girl who has just missed her period" (Castleman 1977, 549). Two months after the bill was originally discussed, the Senate revisited the AHSPPCA's proposal and decided that more information about the issue of teen pregnancy was needed, since discussions of solving the problem had not yet produced a satisfying remedy.

Amid all of the testimony about the AHSPPCA, a majority of those asked to report on teen pregnancy were "expert" witnesses—medical professionals, researchers, or individuals who worked at pregnancy outreach centers. The Senate hearing did include a "teen panel" of four women (all presumably white) who talked about their experiences. One of the women never became pregnant but discussed her experience going to a local clinic to receive contraception to prevent pregnancy, thus fulfilling her obligation as a sexually active teenage girl (Adolescent Health Services [Senate] 1978, 137). The other three witnesses on the panel had had a child during their teenage years. The first of these witnesses married her boyfriend and identified herself as a "wife and mother" (126). Another witness gave her child up for adoption and when asked by senators about her marital and work status admitted to not being married but working for the HEW (for which she was congratulated) (133). A third woman, Valerie Kee, testified about her decision to keep her child, stating that she "planned" to have a child as a teenager but did not know how hard it would be to raise this child on her own. Her testimony emphasizes how she was and still is largely dependent on the Johns Hopkins Center (for teenage mothers). Kee stated that although she was not prepared to have a child, she "was not dumb" because she "knew there was somebody out there that had some backbone" and would offer to help her (136). Throughout her short testimony, Kee returned to the notion that teenagers who do not have support from places like Johns Hopkins are "lost" (not simply in need of support), reinforcing her perception that an intelligent young mother is someone who understands her inherent lack of orientation and identifies an agency that will help her "find" her way through the predicament of teen pregnancy (136). This "panel of teens" ultimately reinforced the goals of the bill as it has been crafted, and the questions they received from senators (e.g., "Have you since married?" "Are you working now?") underscored the shared values of marriage and productivity that informed this preceding (133).

Cynthia Miecznikowski Sheard (1996) contends that epideictic can be an "open" rhetoric, moving "beyond praise and blame," but only if it purposefully concerns itself with the real as well as the "fictive or imaginary—what *might be.*" Such a move enables listeners to extend current beliefs and "envision possible, new, or at least different worlds" (770; emphasis in original). Unfortunately, HEW and Congress did not extend their discussion to how teen pregnancy might be differently understood—perhaps, for example, as an area of concern that implicates males and females, adults and teenagers equally; as a social issue understood in relation to other historical and contemporary shifts in kinship relations; or as an embodied condition that might correlate with some young people already facing adversity that is beyond their control and choice. Perhaps most important, these discussions insisted, directly and indirectly, that teen/unwed pregnancy was unnatural, an abomination and a threat to putatively universal values. The AHSPPCA remained tethered to the closed epideictic of blame that perpetually rendered unwed, pregnant teenage girls "other" and, thus, deficient, their stigmatized bodies the proof of America's declension from the cherished institution of the nuclear family.

Teen Pregnancy, From Public Fear to Private Problem

At a time when many people in the United States believed that the American family was in crisis, the idea of "fixing" a teen pregnancy "problem" seemed to be of unquestionable value. As Eunice Kennedy Shriver told the Senate in her testimony on behalf of the AHSPPCA: "I ask only that you think of this legislation as an essential part of our national commitment to family-building and family-renewal: to the creation of the physical, emotional, and spiritual environment in which the birth of a child and the creation of a family are treated with the respect and reverence they deserve. . . . This troubled, fragile, yet most indispensable of all our human resources is yours to protect" (Adolescent Health Services [Senate] 1978, 125). The late 1970s represented a moment of unparalleled national concern and public discourse related to problematic pregnancy and, thus, an opportunity to (re)shape a national conversation about this public issue in meaningful and constructive ways.

Instead, 1976 to 1980 are years of rhetorical inadequacy in public discussions about helping possible or actual teen mothers—that is, listening to them, supporting them, and working in alliance and in solidarity with them. Circulating discourses that extend from research to public uptake and then to state-directed intervention ultimately make indirect and overdetermined ontological claims that positioned these girls as irredeemably different than the "normal" public and, subsequently, always at odds with public values and goals. That is, public efforts were inadequate in realizing the promise of public intervention, of using congressional deliberation to more fully assess a problem located on some teenage bodies, and of supporting teens in need; all of these possibilities could have come from the response to public fears of a teenage pregnancy epidemic in the form of an epideictic rhetorical approach, which, by definition, calls people together to take action (Hlavacik 2016, 9). What the response to the epidemic of teenage pregnancy did accomplish was undercutting women through blame rhetorics that diminished their character and suggested that they were only "fixable" if understood as infantilized and immature girls. Such a move arrested epistemic possibilities—for publics to reorient to a new moment in reproductive history in ways that expressed care and concern for young women and for women (and men) to cultivate more reproductive knowledge.

This moment of rhetorical inadequacy is responsible for a legacy of blame that deplores unwed pregnancy as lamentable and pins culpability for unwed pregnancy on people who get pregnant, even at the end of a decade of significant change and women's (purportedly, and in important ways, actually) expanding reproductive autonomy. The individual shame of unwed pregnancy thus morphed into a national shame over a perceived surge in teenage sexuality, a pathologizing blame directed at young women, and prioritization of economic values and fears related to capitalism's desire for labor power. Despite the potential for commensurate extensions of youth empowerment and literacy-building, there was little groundswell around discussions that might facilitate such holistic and justice-oriented rethinking. That is, in this moment there was little discursive or policy work that might help people grapple with how young people could be sexual citizens who enjoy (in later reproductive justice framing) the right to have a child, the right to not have a child, and the right to parent in safe and healthy ways. Instead, the nation turned toward young women to rescript righteous reproduction to extend surveillance, limit bodily epistemologies, and curb realistic sexual health literacy. At the same time, the public embrace of this framing arguably bound "teen pregnancy" to poverty in the minds of many people.

The overdetermination of these blame scripts lingers in the minds of many today, so many years later. For instance, a 2012 economic research report on the "uniquely high" rates of teen birth in the United States suggests that the teen pregnancy does not cause poverty (despite this ongoing perception), but instead being poor and "living in a more unequal (and less mobile) location, like the United States, leads young women to choose early, nonmarital childbearing at elevated rates, potentially because of their lower expectations of future economic success" (Kearney and Levine 2012, n.p.). In other words, young pregnant people are not the cause of poverty, nor does such pregnancy determine a subsequent life of poverty. Rather, unjust and unequal systems that withhold social support for some at the benefit of "meritorious" others contribute to bleak futures and prospects of unending precarity—states that do contribute to some young people who are living in poverty choosing parenthood. This is a crucial shift in considering how historical antecedents of personal and social responsibility—the scripts of who is responsible to whom in what ways and for what reasons—have emerged, calcified, and continue into our contemporary moment.

A contrasting opportunity for engaging with young pregnant women is suggested by Wanda, a Black woman who had an unwed pregnancy in 1976 at age 17. Wanda described to me feeling pressured into having sex by a boy who later denied that he was the father of her child. She felt so "dumb" about pregnancy that she did not tell family or friends about her situation, only addressing it fully once she went into labor. Nevertheless, Wanda's best friend visited her at the hospital, congratulated her, assured her that the challenges ahead would be ones she did not need to face alone (despite one of her parents having recently passed), and helped her name her new daughter. Wanda remembers "that day was a turning point for me. I remember saying that I wanted to be a good mother, and I was going to love my baby no matter what her dad did or didn't do. I kept saying in my mind what I had I was going to share it with her." Wanda also recounted her first postbirthing visit with her doctor, someone who was an "inspiration" to her because "he would talk to me about different things and he would talk to me about being a mother and some days it wasn't going to be easy. And some days I wasn't going to know exactly what to do. And that was normal." Even though Wanda spoke to me at length about the more diffuse, if still acute, shame she endured from the birth of her daughter and through many years of being a single mother, these early memories of compassion and shame-countering affirmations offer a glimpse into the rhetorical possibilities for displacing the blame still present at the end of this decade. Indeed, such blame tropes shape public perceptions of teen/unwed pregnancy even today, at a time when debates still continue about how shame is or should be marshalled for the benefit of others.

Conclusion

The Legacies of Righteous Reproduction

Shame as a communicative, rhetorical experience has long lingered, even as it has transformed across decades and in relation to women's also-transforming experiences with reproductive knowledge and sovereignty and in relation to gendered, raced, and classed publicly held norms of righteousness. Analyzing recent past iterations of unsanctioned pregnancy has enabled me to analyze shame's discursive mutations within private and public affective rhetorical ecologies while simultaneously demonstrating how public discourse reflected a perception of shame's dissipation. The paradox of shame's resilience despite claims that it has dissolved (for ill or for good) provides a critical reason for this study; recognizing the power of this emotion, especially in its public instantiations, is a necessary step for those wishing to trace and imagine shame's rhetorical uses and effects. Unbridled, shame can be devastating.[1] Unrecognized and misunderstood, shame can threaten one's sense of political possibility, one's sense of collective possibility, and one's trust in lived experience and embodied epistemologies.

The Value of Historiographic Retelling

This project has retold recent histories of unrighteous reproduction since mid-century in an effort to shed light on histories that have been forgotten, understudied, dismissed, or otherwise not drawn together in an effort to think of them alongside one another and make sense of these linkages. Three findings from this historiographic study are worthy of special attention. First, interweaving various histories of reproduction is a valuable method for understanding and learning from histories of violence and privilege. Additionally, unwed pregnancy as a problem is a rhetorical issue in which responses to perceived fears involve shaming and blaming young women for allegedly unrighteous behavior. And finally, a focus on righteousness and its affective effectuations highlights the rhetorical dangers of upholding cultural logics of durable reproductive progress.

The Value of Telling a More Complete Story

A reverberating silence cloaked the millions of women, most of whom were white, who surrendered a child in the 1950s and 1960s and who continued to experience shame and loneliness in the years after their pregnancy. These women did not forget shame or loss; rather, it remained. Women (white and non-white) who were sterilized against their will also have expressed shame related to that violence. We must bear witness to such stories. We must listen to people who are willing to share them. As Adrienne Rich (1979) explains, "Such themes [of motherhood in bondage] anger and terrify, precisely because they touch us at the quick of human existence. But to flee them, or to trivialize them, to leave the emotions they arouse in us unexamined, is to flee both ourselves and the dawning hope that women *and* men may one day experience forms of love and parenthood, identity and community that will not be drenched in lies, secrets, and silence" (197; emphasis in original).

Part of my work in this book, however, has been to consider a range of experiences that all, in some way, brush against the history of unwed pregnancy. This gathering together of various stories is my attempt to not only *do* the work of recovery but to *do something* with the rhetorical knowledge that comes from such drawing together. By writing feminist rhetorical historiography in light of the lessons of reproductive justice theory and activism, I take up the call by rhetorical scholar Shui-yin Sharon Yam (2020) to make an "overt effort to include, respect, and amplify the voices of marginalized individuals whose reproductive decisions do not conform to white heteronormativity" (32). Yam critiques scholarship in rhetorical studies for primarily examining reproductive rights and focusing "specifically on abortion access and women's rights not to bear children" (20). More analysis of experiences of marginalized people is necessary to extend the work of others, including the rhetorical scholarship of Yam, Natalie Fixmer-Oraiz (2019), and Jenna Vinson. This book has attempted to do such work—both by analyzing unwed and teen pregnancy across several decades and by bringing together stories of women of different races, classes, and social locations.

As a teacher-scholar, I do similar work in bringing together various women's experiences in Rhetorics of Health and Medicine courses that I teach. I have learned from my students the value of attempting to create new awareness from intersectional historiographic study; students help me recognize how, even for those with an interest in women's history and/or women's health, histories are too frequently segregated and delinked in ways that perpetuate ignorance and (for some) sponsor privilege. In a recent graduate course, I had the experience of teaching a group of diverse students (from various humanities and

nonhumanities disciplines; non-white and white, and so on), and our conversations often related to how various aspects of reproductive history and various
raced- and classed-realities of reproductive care are familiar or unfamiliar to
us. After reading about the development of reproductive technologies (as a
cross-racial and cross-class investigation), one white student, Alyssa, writes
that the texts we studied together

> have reignited [my] deep concern for the lack of information provided
> to women of all colors, and particularly white women, regarding the
> problematic history of birth control in the United States. Many of us take
> for granted the success of hormonal manipulation or barrier methods in
> preventing unwanted pregnancies without considering the sacrifices of
> the women whose bodies were appreciated solely for their experimental
> value. We are told that Margaret Sanger was a pioneer in the birth control
> movement, not a racist in her own right. We are offered a plethora of
> contraceptive methods without discussion of the thousands of bodies that
> were abused or butchered in order to bring us the neatly packaged, mod-
> ern pills and devices we use today. Despite having been taught about eu-
> genics previously, it was not until my undergraduate studies in the field of
> biology that I learned about the misuse of hereditary knowledge, and even
> then it was not linked to the development of birth control. The erasure of
> black and brown women from important histories such as these cannot
> continue. There is an uncritical acceptance of medical technology without
> acknowledging the truth about its development, a practice that sheds light
> on our society's lack of empathy and consideration.

I read Alyssa's focus on a dearth of accessible information—"particularly" that
shared with "white women"—not to be a call to recenter the needs of white
students like her but rather a realization of her own sites of ignorance and a
supposition that many other people like her also fail to perceive the interconnectedness of women's recent reproductive history—a site of linkages that cross
lines of race, class, and age. Working with students to consider what histories
are told, which have remained silenced, and how recovery can be an opportunity to engage in historiographic linking across sites of oppression and privilege is valuable because it widens the range of stories shared and thus opens
up space for more possible sharing, more necessary listening (especially among
those who enjoy the privilege of already being listened to and/or heard), and
the vital trust-building that must accompany such efforts. Interlinking enables
perspective-building that also anticipates the yet-unknown and holds space
for future understanding—an openness shared by feminist and reproductive
justice theory. In terms of writing a recent history of enduring shame, my focus on *righteous* reproduction as the framework for the stories shared in this

book has enabled me to attend to scripts of righteousness. These norms—which pregnancies are unsanctioned, when, by whom, and for what reasons—reflect logics undergirding much of the shifting affective rhetorical ecologies related to and the material practices enacted on reproducing bodies in recent decades.

Unwed Pregnancy as (in Part) a
Rhetorical Problem of "Othered" Bodies

Rhetorics of shame—radial rhetorics of private shame, stigmatizing rhetorics of contagious bodily shame, sticky rhetorics of persistent shame, and shifting rhetorics of shame-expressed-as-blame—are an indisputable feature of the stories of unwed pregnancy during the era of hiding and surrender and the long 1970s. The rhetorics manifest during these years shifted to meet the demands of rapidly changing rhetorical situations. But what did not change was the way in which these rhetorical depictions always rendered unwed pregnancy to be some sort of problem, albeit a problem differently defined at various times and with disparate ramifications. Fears led to efforts to protect what was variously configured to be righteous and valuable: the white heteronormative family, the school, the authority of male-centered institutions, the economic interests of the US taxpayer, the young and innocent white child who could be rehabilitated. This problematic view of unwed pregnancy, and later teen pregnancy, is persistently focused on women's bodies as a site of deviance and abnormality.

What stops one from naturalizing unwed or teen pregnancy, given the fact that such "conditions" are only possible given the "natural" capabilities of many—if not all—human bodies? A normalizing discussion of sexuality is largely missing from these conversations. A historical and cultural obsession with sexual norms and the rhetorical performance of pregnancy as it is socially sanctioned—as righteous reproduction—overrides the ability to talk about such forms of pregnancy as typical and contextual, even if not in all cases ideal or desirable. This cultural habituation toward viewing unwed- or teen-pregnancy-as-problem functions as what Kenneth Burke (1965) describes as a "trained incapacity," or "the state of affairs whereby one's very abilities" can prevent accurately or fully comprehending a situation (7). The long tradition of rhetorically constructing unwed pregnancy as a problematic, abnormal, and shameful state continues to function as a trained incapacity (what Burke also refers to as *blindness*, using problematically ableist language); such incapacities preclude recognizing, understanding, and deliberating about unwed and teen pregnancy in more productive or nuanced ways—and in conversation with the people who are living or have lived this experience. By employing historiography of the recent past, this book attempts to contribute to the important rhetorical work—especially that of Vinson, Fixmer-Oraiz (2019), and Yam—being done to center the experiences of marginalized reproducing women.

This project also demonstrates the pervasiveness of the sexual double standard within the recent history of unwed pregnancy. Of the numerous primary texts I have encountered during this research, a paltry few consider unwed or teenage pregnancy as a "problem" faced by two people who had sexual intercourse. Overwhelmingly, and to disturbing and infuriating ends, unwed and teen pregnancy is rhetorically constructed as being a female problem. Discussions of unwed and teen pregnancy most frequently do not address the unwed father, although when they do it is often to suggest that unwed mothers use a pregnancy to "trap" a man into marriage (a trope that seems not to have faded away over the years). What's more, some of the women I interviewed who surrendered their child for adoption were strongly encouraged or forced to list the father as "unknown" on their child's birth certificate, even when the father was known—a practice that ostensibly lessened the threat of a father attempting to claim paternity, which might slow down or reverse adoption arrangements. Through the 1960s and the long 1970s, women and girls "got themselves in trouble" while men and boys avoided the gendered shame and stigma of sex outside of marriage. In sum, unwed and teen pregnancy remained a mistake, and a female one at that. The legal, verbal, and visual rhetorics perpetuating this idea contributed to the delegitimization and vilification of unwed mothers.

Despite these sites of enduring discourses and logics, a rhetorical approach to examining sites of injustice creates space for engaging with history and pursuing rhetorical reconfiguration. For instance, it is easy to perpetuate shaming practices by engaging with history and (simply) identifying perpetrators and victims. The more valuable work is to engage in deep contextualization to understand how arguments and suasive affects made sense to original audiences and how they led to material effects. The malleability of rhetoric means that past ideas must be interrogated with contextual rigor (even if they are not fully exonerated or explained away as "just the way things were").

Rhetoric's plasticity is also a reminder of its possibility. For instance, the National Crittenton, the current iteration of the Florence Crittenton Mission chartered in 1893, has reenvisioned its work toward justice, using advocacy and activism to "ensure that girls and gender-expansive young people have the support and opportunities they need to heal, be safe, be free, and experience joy." According to the organization's website and my discussion with Jeannette Pai-Espinosa, the current president, National Crittenton has considered the value that could be drawn from the earliest iterations of its work, has openly acknowledged its role in wider cultural practices of "going away," and has identified how it can move forward to address a range of types of adversity experienced by young people—but letting the "wisdom of cis and trans girls, young women, and gender-expansive young people of color" lead these varied efforts. The organization is an exemplar of the possibilities of rhetorical reconfiguration—work that does not operate from a logic of blame or defensiveness but instead with the goals of radically reshaping and reimagining what justice looks like and how to achieve it.

The Danger in Upholding Cultural Logics
of Reproductive Progress

"It used to be called illegitimacy. Now it is the new normal." This claim opens a front-page *New York Times* article on unwed motherhood published in February 2012. The article continues: "After steadily rising for five decades, the share of children born to unmarried women has crossed a threshold: more than half of births to American women under thirty occur outside marriage" (DeParle and Tavernise 2012). Although social, political, and economic contexts change, unwed pregnancy long has been and will long continue to be a reality in the United States. The complex history of unwed pregnancy reflects how this "problem" is one that is always tied to women's social identity, worth, and rhetorical power—a power that emanates from their pregnant bodies and constrains or enables them to speak, to be spoken for, and to be listened to or ignored. Even as times and trends change, the term *unwed mother* continues to be saturated with meaning that has accumulated over time. Because so many of those meanings are unspoken but invoked by the pregnant body, giving voice to such rhetorical baggage is of historical and contemporary importance.

Across my early interviews, I was surprised to hear why the women with whom I spoke wanted to share their story of hiding and surrender. Although some women are still working through their own grief and sense of betrayal, others warned that they wanted to talk about their experiences as unwed mothers because they worried our society might return to the seemingly outdated ways of thinking inflicted upon them and captured in their stories. *Send women away to maternity homes? Force them to relinquish their child? Shame them into secrecy?* I silently posed these questions to myself in disbelief. *How could that happen? Surely that could not really happen again!* I listened, but I was not convinced that sharing stories of unwed pregnancy was of dire need *now,* in relation to contemporary culture and politics. I did however (and still do) have a firm commitment that this portion of women's history should be given fuller attention, especially given the systematic silencing of unwed mothers and other poor and/or potentially multiply marginalized women who have experienced reproductive violence. When I first read Ann Fessler's (2007) *The Girls Who Went Away,* I was shocked that this history happened, that it happened during the lifetime of my parents and the adults who shaped my youth, and that I (someone particularly interested in women's history) had never previously heard about it. I was skeptical of the warning these mothers shared, although I respected their opinions. After all, they had gone away. They had relinquished the child they carried to term. They lived all of this, and I did not.

In the process of researching and composing this project, however—in the years before the election of Donald Trump and before the confirmations of Justice Brett Kavanaugh and Justice Amy Coney Barrett to the US Supreme Court (the latter happening after the death of Justice Ruth Bader Ginsberg), events that many nonconservatives point to as an indication of regression in feminist gains of recent decades—I began to have my own doubts about the assuredness of reproductive political "gains." Learning from reproductive justice activism and scholarship and from my original research helped me to more fully comprehend how slowly and unevenly (when at all) basic rights were afforded to women in relation to their reproductive capacities. I realized my own unchecked belief in the power of the *Roe* decision, for example, to mark a permanent turning point in women's reproductive history. Learning about the rhetorical efforts of people like Clydie Marie Perry, Byllye Avery, Barbara Seaman, Katsi Cook, and Bill Baird illuminated just how strong and pervasive resistance was to women's ability to attend school when pregnant, to read safety and product information about the oral contraceptives that they were taking, to understand their bodies as sites of colonial violence and resistance, and to talk to a doctor about birth control irrespective of their marital status. All in all, change was incremental. It was met with resistance based on stubborn cultural logics about unwed pregnancy, the sexual double standard, and righteous dependency that lingered and always circled back to the assumption that some person other than the woman in question could better speak for her sexual and reproductive needs and desires.

When I compare these hard-fought efforts with the pervasiveness and sheer endurance of a sexual double standard that holds people with uteruses primarily accountable for all types of sexual encounters and their outcomes, I realize that women's gains in recent history are laudable but certainly not unshakeable or irreversible. Much of the same misogynistic *doxa* of the early part of the twentieth century that I touch upon in chapter 1 still held sway in the 1960s and the 1970s, and such beliefs continue to shape expectations about sex today. Such longevity encourages recognizing the extent to which women's claims over their bodies are fragile and the extent to which supremacy endures, assuming various iterations but always advancing hierarchies based on distinctions between purported normalcy and non-normate bodies. This finding sounds simple and straightforward, but if it were, then reproductive justice would be an effort of the past. Nevertheless, it becomes easy to lull oneself into the disbelief that the past is the past—that current times are different, current publics (at least those aligned with one's values) more enlightened.

Unpacking the cultural logics of righteous notions of reproduction can enable us to push back against ways of thinking that erroneously perpetuate a sense of "evolutionary historical progress" (Ratcliffe 2019, 42). Such evolutionary thinking—evident in the macrochange narratives I examined in chapter 3—encourages people to believe that women's reproductive freedoms have consistently expanded, that all women have significant levels of reproductive choice, and that shame related to reproduction and sexuality is mostly a vestige of earlier, less "civilized" times—such as times when white unwed mothers "went away." But as the stories of this book have suggested, such evolutionary thinking can not only be inaccurate but can fuel new emotions, such as worry and anger over a seemingly new era of reproductive political "rollbacks." While people *should* be vigilant and responsive to violations of reproductive justice of any kind, it is just as critical to pursue education about "women's" progress by considering the perspective of various people based on their lived experiences and tracing how protections have extended (or not) to them.

Krista Ratcliffe has recently expanded her notion of cultural logic, originally described in *Rhetorical Listening: Identification, Gender, Whiteness,* so as to explicitly apply it to gender politics. Ratcliffe (2019) reminds us that a cultural logic is "a way of reasoning common to a group of people, a way of reasoning that changes over time and place" (42). The power of cultural logics, Ratcliffe contends, is that they "influence significations of words functioning as tropes" (42). Frustrated with how the 2012 US election cycle seemed to reflect a moment of backlash against feminist gains and a so-called war on women, Ratcliffe channeled her affective energies into an attempt to critique her own expectations of progress. She explains the cultural logic of gender politics that she was beholden to as follows:

- *If* we assume that each generation evolves ever upward by becoming healthier, wealthier, and wiser,
- *then* we believe that women's political and economic gains (that have resulted from hard-fought cultural debates) emerge as a stable base . . . ,
- *therefore,* we conclude that the stable base ensures current rights and future gains for women. (42; emphasis in original)

The logic of gender-oriented political progress that Ratcliffe maps can apply to righteous reproduction as well; we only need to substitute "reproductive" gains for those advances listed above and think about how "choice" is one such trope that relies on this flawed logic. This logic, when considered alongside the persistent, sticky, and shape-shifting quality of gendered sexual shame that is so fully part of many women's lived reproductive realities, warrants the careful and ongoing study of reproductive histories in service of a more robust and intersectional awareness of where we (all) have been, where we are now, and where we are going.

These conclusions help to explain why unwed pregnancy during recent decades has been misunderstood and even overlooked by scholars and the general public alike. Too frequently seen as the source of a problem, unwed mothers have been historically marginalized—shamed, blamed, silenced, and even ignored while being the focus of intervention. Examining the rhetorics that constrain these mothers' voices—at the time of their pregnancy and, for some, long after—enables historiographic research and, hopefully, engenders further study and activism.

Using Affective Awareness: What's to Be Done with Shame?

New York Times opinion columnist Bret Stephens has recently labeled the era of former President Donald Trump a time of the "annihilation of shame." Penning a nostalgic take on "days bygone" in which behaving properly, feeling remorse, and being penitent was an ostensibly appropriate response to shame, Stephens (2019) designates a "Trumpian method of avoiding shame," which is "not giving a damn." He continues: "Spurious bone-spur draft deferment? Shrug. Fraudulent business and charitable practices? Snigger. Outrageous personal invective? Sneer. Inhumane treatment of children at the border? Snarl. Hush-money payoffs to porn-star and centerfold mistresses? Stud!" Stephens argues that along with President Trump's impudence, public acquiescence allows for a contemporary moment that lacks the regulatory function—the useful public role—of shame. And even though Trump served only as a one-term president, his legacy (especially in terms of the three US Supreme Court justices confirmed during his presidency) as well as the ongoing resonance of his unapologetic shamelessness as a form of toxic masculinity will, at least for now, endure. Trump channels rage and victimization as a form of white, male, cisgender, ableist, and heteronormative virtuousness, and his followers embrace and ostensibly adopt for themselves his shamelessness, ire, and desire for vengeance (Kelly 2019).

Trump's disavowal of feeling shame, an emotion so linked to victimhood and vulnerability, suggests another slippery uptake of the emotion: selectively ignoring it is a performance of toughness, but doing so also implicitly values its existence as contributing to white, male supremacist culture in the United States. Significantly, a tolerance of shame should not be taken for granted but should, instead, be understood as a desire for a return to shame. Jill Locke (2016) theorizes what she refers to as "the lament that shame is dead," or a "nostalgic story of an imagined past that represents a longing for a mythical place and time when shame secured and regulated social life" (18). According to Locke, the lament is powerful in framing good citizenship and sharpest when ordinary people, "especially those lacking significant political power and status, resist and refashion the demands of shame and its requirements" (20). The call for a return to shame, then, is an effort to gird against the perceived chaos of an imagined culture of shamelessness, a surfeit of unaccountable personal freedoms.

Locke's (2016) contention that shame is nonontological and instead "discursively and corporeally produced" underscores the value of tracing its rhetorical migration; she posits that shame actually manifests through discussions of what it is, where it is located, and—frequently—its apparent demise, which is referenced as a sign of civic and moral decline (19). She also warns against a recuperation of shame as a "normative emotion to be cultivated to steer and salvage democratic life and democratic equality" because shame operates through a perpetual practice of self- and other-directed surveillance (34). Additionally, calls to rise above shame through proclamations of dignity and unabashed pride fetishize a political economy that operates beyond shame's reach. In terms resonant with this book, such attempts to deny shame threaten to ignore shame's sometimes surreptitious presence and its contributions to reinscribing righteousness. A world reeling from the experiences of the global COVID-19 pandemic has dealt with—and will likely again deal with—the vexing questions of shame's perceived utility in times of contagion and in ways that often leverage extant sentiments of difference, hierarchy, and xenophobia.

How should feminists orient themselves to shame, then, given its long-standing interconnectedness with processes of feminization and the violences that it performs as a method for normalizing as this study of reproductive righteousness has shown? What role does or should shame play in ongoing publicity related to women's sexual and reproductive lives? Do these questions intensify in light of its uptake in other contexts of perceived or real (i.e., social or biological) contagion? In short, how should shame, rhetorically speaking, be valued today by those advocating from marginalized positions given a hypermediated, politically polarized, and—for many—dangerous landscape?

These are complex questions that I cannot fully answer. This book lays out a recent history of righteous reproduction in an effort to perform the work of tracing shame's appearances and mutations from a recent past that informs (but also that fails to sufficiently inform) reproductive politics today. Anyone who cares about reproductive issues will benefit from learning more complete recent histories and from seeking out stories that mitigate partial and privileged knowledges that uphold the injustice of righteousness. At the same time, we can continue to identify righteous reproduction today by using our attunement to rhetoric, feminism, and reproductive justice theory to ask how it materializes, what its current economies are, who calls upon it, and how is it called upon.

I use this final meditation and a particular case study to argue that shame, while being weaponized by various actors to disrupt ongoing sites of violence and silencing, still operates in a closed rhetorical system. This closed system—one that is bound to the interrelationship of both shame and honor—fails to effectively reconfigure power dynamics even as it points to abuses of power in order to critique them. Shame, still insufficiently misunderstood as rhetorical, thus threatens to thwart change and healing when it is used in service of political and social justice. Like Locke, I am dubious of efforts to use shame for liberatory purposes, although my particular rationale stems from my skepticism of shame's ability to ultimately break a normalizing ecology. The story of Maddi Runkles, a high school senior who became pregnant in 2017 and was subsequently dismissed from her Christian school, offers an illustration of this assertion.

Shame in a New Key: The Case of Maddi Runkles

In May 2017, the story of Madeline "Maddi" Runkles made headlines around the country. Runkles, a white student who was poised to graduate from Heritage Academy, a private Christian pre-kindergarten through grade 12 school in Hagerstown, Maryland, was barred from walking in the school's graduation ceremony because she was pregnant. I briefly recount the story of Runkles's presence in the media not only because she represents a contemporary instance of unrighteous reproduction (to some) because of her unwed pregnancy but because shame figures so powerfully in her story of dismissal and, later, her *ethos* for those who uplifted her as being an emblem of reproductive virtue. I use Runkles's story to provide a contemporary example of shame's mutability. I close this chapter by noting the danger of weaponizing shame and by suggesting ways that feminist scholars might warn against unjust (if unintentional) applications of shame and imagine and amplify rhetorical strategies for operating outside the pale of shame altogether.

Runkles (2017) opens a piece she pens for the *Washington Post* with the unflinching admission that she will "have a baby boy as a result of my deliberate failure to adhere to a pledge of chastity I signed at my school." Starting in grade five, Heritage Academy students are expected to comply with a nine-part "statement of faith," a portion of which dictates that "no intimate sexual activity be engaged in outside of the marriage commitment between a man and woman" (quoted in Stolberg 2017). Runkles, age 18 by the time of graduation, was an unmarried mother-to-be and thus exemplified to Heritage Academy a defiance of the school's sexual purity code. According to Heritage Academy principal Dave Hobbs, "Even though we love Maddi, even though we forgive her, there's still accountability" based on Runkles's "breach of the standard of abstinence" (quoted in Wright and Hawkins 2017). In a media interview, Hobbs added that such a violation "is a grievous choice" that "Maddi made" (quoted in Heim 2017). "Forgiveness," Hobbs explained, "does not mean there's no accountability" (quoted in Heim 2017).

Accountability for breaking a chastity pledge becomes a vexing goal when one person (a woman) is held to a standard that was broken privately, through action that somehow involved another person (here, a man), and that results in life being created. In a letter to parents days before the graduation ceremony, Hobbs attempted to draw some lines of clarification. He shared that the school punished Runkles "not because she is pregnant but because she was immoral," and instructed that "the best way to love her right now is to hold her accountable for her morality that began this situation" (quoted in Heim 2017). Thus, Runkles's supposed intent, not the effects of her "choice" required punishment. When, in another statement to NBC News, Hobbs claimed that Heritage Academy was "being bullied" based on expanding coverage of and controversy over the story, the principal asked the network to "please tell America that we are not disciplining Maddi because she chose to keep her baby boy . . . For that, we commend her" (Yoder 2017).

Before this story garnered media attention, Runkles faced immediate punishment for her "transgression": she was suspended for two days while the school board decided on further action (Wright and Hawkins 2017). Runkles's father, Scott, was serving as the head of the school board at the time. He initially recused himself from decisions related to Maddi and later resigned from the board based on Maddi's treatment (Stolberg 2017). The school's first set of additional punishments included Runkles being suspended, stripped of her title as student council president and other leadership positions, barred from all sporting events, uninvited to campus until after giving birth, made to finish her senior year coursework at home, and deemed ineligible to walk in the Heritage Academy graduation ceremony (Heim 2017; Runkles 2017). After the Runkles family appealed to the school board on the basis of the severity and unparalleled quality of this punishment (as compared to other violations of the school honor code), Heritage Academy altered the punishment so that Maddi could attend school through the end of the year. She was still prohibited from maintaining her leadership positions and from walking at graduation (Runkles 2017). According to Maddi's mother Sharon, some teachers stopped acknowledging her daughter; a rumor circulated that the principal had asked some teachers to have Maddi sit in the rear of the classroom (Wright and Hawkins 2017). And according to Maddi, community members who initially supported her once she "went public" took a different tack once attention was drawn to Heritage Academy. "We started getting nasty emails, angry posts on social media and rude remarks in person. People who had been supportive before are now telling me to shut up, suck it up and grow up." Citing the "volume of anger from the community," Runkles notes that her parents decided that both she and her brother would finish the school year from home. Runkles's takeaway: others considered her to be "attention-seeking and spoiled" (Heim 2017). Runkles was too visible (i.e., public) as a pregnant student to be at school and too public (i.e., desirous of visibility) in her appeal for equality.

At some point during this period—or as Maddi states, "on top of all of this" (Runkles 2017), Hobbs decided to hold a school assembly to inform all Heritage Academy students (and their families, who were invited to also attend) of the situation.[2] Hobbs did not want Maddi to attend the assembly, but she "volunteered" to be there and asked to personally speak to the student body. According to Maddi, "I was a senior and a campus leader, so I felt as if I should tell them myself" (Runkles 2017). Maddi explains the event from her point of view: "In front of the whole school, I got up and started to read a statement I wrote explaining that I had broken the rules, that I was repentant and that I asked for forgiveness. But I couldn't get through it. My dad had to read some of it while I composed myself. It was one of the hardest things I ever did, and I'm so sorry, not for myself but for any girl in that audience who will get pregnant in the future and may consider abortion because of what I had to go through." This recounting of her own experience cuts to the heart of the controversy that Runkles's pregnancy—and her pregnant body—represented to US culture in 2017. Her story ricocheted though news outlets not as a salacious tale of teen passion but as a reincarnation of scarlet letter-style public shaming. It read as a performance meant to demonstrate allegiance to purity while simultaneously threatening to disincentivize other young pregnant women from keeping a child, should they have to endure such public judgment. The right to have a child and the right to not have a child were dangerously intermingled in and on Runkles.

The attention this story generated initially suggests its value as a site of rhetorical examination, as does its inability to align neatly with partisan and ideological divides related to, for instance, sex education and abortion politics. Additionally, it is true that Heritage Academy's choice and approach of sharing information about Runkles's pregnancy as well as its subsequent informal and official disciplining of her conforms to the claim made by Vinson (2018) that "the argument to prevent teenage pregnancy functions on the stigmatization and surveillance of young women" (xiv). I see value in thinking about young women's experiences of being surveilled regarding reproductive choices across sacred and secular communities, and I have been intrigued, surprised, and not surprised to witness the white and relatively affluent Runkles function as a material-discursive fulcrum for an impassioned, if brief, national story about reproduction. The emotional characterization of, interest in, and varied response to Runkles's situation evidences that her school's attempt to hide her from graduation backfired—that, as an echo of that older practice of hiding, such a punishment is perceived as antiquated and, thus, as a new take on hiding it functioned as the true source of shame.

Advocacy on behalf of Runkles—advocacy that is central to this story breaking as national news—articulates an honor-shame order whereby Heritage Academy figures as shameful in its treatment of Runkles as a visibly pregnant student. This ongoing advocacy reverses the honor-shame order so as to "reembody" Runkles as a courageous and autonomous reproductive agent. Here I borrow the term *reembody* from Nathan Stormer (2004), who uses it to describe a process of "coming to have a public voice" (267) within his larger exploration of articulation—or connection—and *taxis* to identify "performative regime[s]" of "linguistic and embodied interconnections, or articulations" (261). Such figuration of Runkles leverages the persuasive power of choice feminism and illustrates an effort to articulate *choice*, a term typically associated with reproductive autonomy but that is disavowed within a reproductive justice frame, with obedience to a pronatalist and anti-abortion ideology.

Runkles reports having reached out to Students for Life of America after having disclosed her pregnancy to see if the organization could "use [her] story to help other girls" (Students for Life of America [SFLA] 2017, "Autumn's"). A pro-life group, SFLA exists to "recruit, train, and mobilize the pro-life generation to abolish abortion" (SFLA 2017, "About"). SFLA and its president Kristan Hawkins soon became part of Runkles's story; Hawkins acted as a sort of spokesperson alongside Runkles during public and media appearances and SFLA was a key organizer for a graduation ceremony and was a donor supporting the graduate's forthcoming enrollment at Bob Jones University. Runkles subsequently spoke for SFLA—specifically at an anti-abortion rally in Washington, DC. Notably, it is Hawkins as advocate and activist who initially and most provocatively invokes shame in speaking of Heritage Academy's response to Runkles. Hawkins notes that Runkles's situation raises a "question a lot of Christian schools have to grapple with, holding our students to high standards and expecting them to practice chastity before marriage . . . But then, also, how do we love those who become pregnant and how do we not shame them?" She more pointedly asked of Hobbs's actions: "Why would you call an all-school assembly, inviting students, parents, and faculty and say you're going to announce to the entire school the sins of one student?" (Wright and Hawkins 2017).

The shaming that Hawkins points to relies on a moralistic order that is upheld by a discursive commitment to chastity as well as through the visibility of nonpregnant bodies (or the invisibility of pregnant bodies). Hawkins's regular use of the term *shame* when speaking of the situation makes it a centerpiece of the narrative. The blame that SFLA levels at the school for its lack of

Christian sympathy, then, succeeds in demonstrating the school's articulation of Runkles's sexual and reproducing body to the putative "sin" of premarital sex. The pregnant body that decades ago threatened a family through shame's perceived radial contagion now threatens a private, religious school committed to purity. Significantly, the school's pursuit of purity functions as a zero-sum game: evidence of sin detracts from the honor of the institution. Hawkins suggests that the school assembly was meant to locate sin on Runkles as a sexual and reproducing body and thus reassert the school's purity. Through this suggestion, she also implies that Runkles's mothering body is not of concern to the school and that Runkles-as-pregnant teenager does not receive sufficient love, mercy, or protection from the institution. Further, SFLA's visual and verbal advocacy for Runkles functions as a material-discursive act that reembodies this pregnant-while-unmarried-Christian woman. Instead of being rendered invisible, Runkles appears publicly in new and different ways as suggested by the images of her that circulated publicly: Runkles alongside Hawkins on Fox News, beside Hawkins and behind a giant SFLA donation check, with her diploma and in her cap-and-gown while pregnant.[3]

Runkles's story not only resulted in her portrayal as a victim of an unjust school; significantly, she emerges as a courageous young woman, an exemplar of reproductive choice, and an emblem for pro-life activists. Runkles casts herself in this light when she writes about her experience for the *Washington Post*: "When girls like me who go to pro-life schools make a brave pro-life decision, we shouldn't be hidden away in shame. The sin that got us into this situation is not worth celebrating, but after confession and forgiveness take place we should be supported and treated like any other student. What we are going through is tough enough. Having to deal with the added shame of being treated like an outcast is nothing that any girl should have to go through" (Runkles 2017). This depiction of Runkles as a willful and brave individual standing up for morality against adversity echoes through the various commentaries about her; the traction of her story, it seems, was her sympathetic position as well as her ability to follow her convictions despite the shaming she knew she would likely endure.

Contributing to this narrative of courageousness is Runkles's own admission that she contemplated getting an abortion (even though she is an avowed pro-life Christian) because she anticipated the judgment that would be passed on her by others in her community. And her decision to appear in front of the school contributes to a climate of shaming that she faced head-on. While there is no doubt that this public confession necessitated personal fortitude, as a self-flagellant testimony, it simultaneously reifies the perceived shamefulness of women who "choose" to have intercourse outside of marriage. In other words, Runkles feels the need to make her statement a confession, to publicly recommit herself to ideological/religious purity through an explicit refusal to quietly obtain an abortion and, ostensibly, invisibly perform a type of revirginalization through nondisclosure. In a *New York Times* article, she shares that she "told on" herself, "asked for forgiveness," and "asked for help" (Stolberg 2017)—all discursive moves that highlight her position of interdependency and her interest in upholding a code of virtue that inhibits sexual sovereignty, acceptance, and expression.

Runkles's courageousness—and the uptake of her courage narrative by pro-life groups—relies precisely on her exercising her right to have a child and parent that child with dignity—two reproductive justice values. Conversely, a woman in her situation who exercises her right to not have a child may or may not find similar support. Despite notable efforts to the contrary (such as using #shoutyourabortion as a strategy to galvanize anti-shaming stories on social media), the decision to have an abortion is infrequently shared or understood as an act of bravery or, less exceptionally, as an act that people have made through history in light of their personal assessment of their needs, capabilities, and desires at the time of pregnancy. Additionally, Hawkins undercuts claims of sovereignty as beneficial by claiming that Planned Parenthood disempowers women and encourages abortion because teenagers are not "strong enough" to choose life (SFLA 2017, "Martha"). In this way, a particular type of agency—pro-life reproductive sovereignty—becomes the basis of praise in part through casting abortion as a shameful, uninformed choice of the weak.

In reversing an honor-shame order to take shame away from this young woman, a zero-sum equation—namely, the closed rhetorical system of shame—still applies. Shame does not disappear; rather, it becomes reassigned. Similar to Emily Winderman's concept of "volume" to explain the regulation of another emotion—anger—when dispatched from rhetors enjoying or being denied privilege, shame's rhetorical and affective effectuation in public has serious implications as it courses across rhetorical landscapes. But whereas Winderman (2019) concludes that anger is "available for some to mobilize while simultaneously limiting the emotional expression—and thus the political potential—of others" (329), I would argue that public shame largely resists regulation and can be easily weaponized by those in various positions related to power in an effort to silence.

Runkles's story suggests how contemporary rhetorics of reproduction and contested motherhood are expressions of righteousness that reveal shame newly placed but still present. It also provides a window onto activism among young women that is premised on non–justice-oriented allegiances to choice (a key trope of evolutionary reproductive politics) and a belief in autonomy even when that autonomy is beholden to some honor-shame order. Maddi Runkles and her baby's invitation to meet with former Vice President Pence and Mrs.

Pence suggests the signifying power of reproducing people who articulate to righteousness. Runkles continues to function as a material-discursive fulcrum of consequence and a powerful site of persuasion for activists committed to influencing women's reproductive capabilities.

Final Thoughts: Beyond Writing Shame

Runkles's story illustrates that shame's potency and mutability renders it able to be deployed and redirected to unexpected ends. With this consideration in mind, I conclude by revisiting recent efforts to better account for the value of writing shame and the limitations or oversights of such valuable rhetorical shame theory.

The #MeToo movement offers new ways to think about rhetoric, sexual shame, and notions of righteousness, even though it requires a pivot from issues of reproduction to concerns about sexual violence and the cultures and economies of shame that enable such aggression and assault. Shari J. Stenberg (2018) argues that shame can function as a site of "revisionary work" (120) and that *writing shame* (a term she borrows from Elspeth Probyn) can be an "invitational, critical, and generative rhetorical act" (121). Stenberg reaches this conclusion after studying tweets created by people sharing their first assaults and using the hashtag #NotOkay. This outpouring of personal accounts made public came in the wake of the release of an *Access Hollywood* recording in which Donald Trump boasted about his ability to sexually assault women due to his celebrity status. Author and public figure Kelly Oxford invited women to "tweet her their first assaults," resulting in more than 27 million responses (Stenberg 2018, 120). Stenberg focuses on how this invitation to disclose helped women trust that they would be believed if they shared their story and thus resisted "shaming practices" that typically result in silencing (126). She also contends that the emotions described in tweets help to explain the emotional landscape of feelings—such as shame and grief—that typically dissuade survivors of sexual assault from speaking through shame to share their story. The tweets also call attention to the cultural structures and belief systems, such as rape culture, that enable such shaming to take place (128). This study of writing shame is useful in helping to imagine ways that shame can be accounted for and resisted in public. Stenberg's work aligns with Dianna Taylor's (2018) call for "feminist innovation specifically concerning solidarity"—a coalitional effort to rupture the logics of individuation inherent to gendered shame through "collective, inclusive, public, [and] corporal practices" that allow women to create "counter-normalizing modes of constituting, understanding, and relating to ourselves" (447). Shame's social qualities can, in certain instances, help move people from feelings of self-rejection and isolation and into coalition; both feminist scholars suggest the benefits of doing just that.

But I would also argue that group practices of leveraging, mobilizing, and deploying shame can undercut feminist values (such as the immanent worth of all humans) when amplified as happens, for instance, in so-called cancel culture. Here I am referring to contemporary practices of trying to "cancel" or "culturally" block a person from enjoying a prominent career or place in the public eye (Romano 2019). At the time of my writing, this term itself is being weaponized; claims of the injustice of ideologically driven "cancelling" are steeped in partisan practices of defensiveness and toxic victimhood that also silence in that they functionally resist efforts to listen, understand, and work coalitionally toward human rights and justice for all people. According to Anne Charity Hudley, canceling has long been part of Black culture and has been part of the empowerment and civil rights movements (Romano 2019). Cancel culture is a practice of public shaming that is similar to, often confused with, but arguably different than call-out culture—giving voice to shameful acts or beliefs through expressions of shame, or shame communicated to another person or entity. Both cancel culture and call-out culture are especially present on social media, where virality can render someone not only called-out in a very public way but, potentially, cancelled.

Survivors may need to rely on shaming to name perpetrators as a necessary measure for stopping abuse and actively seeking safety and healing; I wish to honor this use of shame as explained by movement mediator adrienne maree brown (2020). In relation to other instances of harm and injustice that are less explicitly connected to personal safety (a potentially murky distinction, to be sure), it might be promising for those who have been silenced to deploy shame. ("Shame on you!" is an exclamation I often see in public writing, such as on social media.) This expression sometimes seems to be spectacle-producing; it is meant to call attention to some wrong and to make the recipient being called out feel bad and be seen feeling bad. And as Jodi Nicotra (2016) explains, when such public shaming takes place online—and especially in "hyper-circulatory" spaces such as Twitter—it not only "performatively" enacts "norms and values" but builds community. But as Runkles's experience suggests, rhetors have little control over how shame might be redeployed and how it might linger and reappear in new and unanticipated ways. The closed rhetorical system of communicated shame that I suggest above operates within a shame-honor continuum that doesn't seem to dissolve shame. A resurgence in what one might call *teflon toxic masculinity* means that anti-feminist public figures choose not to register the effects of weaponized shaming. In such a context, this strategy of deploying shame as an attack seems futile in changing minds and hearts, even if it supports feelings of catharsis and solidarity building among the aggrieved.

Several public voices contribute meaningfully to these vexed ideas about shame's uses. Reproductive justice activist Loretta J. Ross has expressed her reservations about call-out and cancel-culture as communication methods that can support justice. Considering how publics can "hold each other accountable while doing extremely difficult and risky social justice work," Ross (2019) urges readers to understand the danger in "individualizing oppression" and using movement as "personal therapy space." In expressing her concern over the unexamined consequences of public shaming, Ross—a self-identified victim of sexual abuse—argues, "I believe #MeToo survivors can more effectively address sexual abuse without resorting to the punishment and exile that mirror the prison industrial complex. Nor should we use social media to rush to judgment in a courtroom composed of clicks. If we do, we run into the paradox Audre Lorde warned us about when she said that 'the master's tools will never dismantle the master's house.'" Ross further warns that the act of calling out cultivates the fear that one will be targeted. She even discloses her own experience of having "froze[n] in shame" when accidentally misgendering a student when teaching. Ross's insights help to show the danger of deployments of shame, even if they are taken up in the spirit of justice.

brown (2020), whose careful work to contemplate canceling as "punitive justice" (41) should be read in full, also suggests a "social destruction" (40) in shame-based movement culture. Naming call outs as acts that "elicit both a consistent negative and dismissive energy, and a pleasurable take-down activation, regardless of what the call out is addressing" (26), brown attends to the multiple affects mixed up in punitive shaming. Fear is, as Ahmed suggests, borne in the contact between surfaces. An unrighteous contact—whether intentional or not (such as in the case of accidental misgendering) is to be feared; the policing of such contact is what fuels a culture of public shame. Such shame deployment is weaponized not as much to actually promote knowledge-making, knowledge-sharing, and healing but to provide a cathartic reaction— a release of anger or hurt. Therefore, while I am hopeful that there will continue to be opportunities to write shame in ways that shed light on what might otherwise remain unspoken, I also argue that feminists must more fully contend with vexing relationships to shame, particularly in ways that are not only based in testimony but that involve expressions of casting shame on others. Although it might not be directed primarily (or perhaps at all) to someone like me, brown's vision of movement, justice, and abolition imagined beyond shame is instructive. "We won't end the systemic patterns of harm by isolating and picking off individuals, just as we can't limit the communicative power of mycelium by plucking a single mushroom from the dirt. We need to flood the entire system with life-affirming principles and practices, to clear the channels between us of the toxicity of supremacy, to heal from the harms of a legacy of devaluing some lives and needs in order to indulge others" (8). I agree with brown that communicating shame through call outs fails at the critical work of "addressing misunderstandings, issuing critiques, or resolving contradiction" (46).

Shame has been purposefully communicated or purposefully withheld as part of centuries-old practices of designating levels of humanity (on the basis of race and class) and registering the capability of being righteous. As Tessa McWatt (2020) reminds, shame is one of a variety of classificatory schemes that has designated worth: "Influenced by a taxonomy of human beings introduced in *Systema Naturae,* first published in 1735 by Swedish botanist, zoologist and physician Carl Linnaeus, philosophers and naturalists began to make scientific distinctions among humans. Linneaus's succinct classification of the African '*Afer* or *Africanus*' consisted of 'black, phlegmatic, relaxed. *Hair* black, frizzled. *Skin* silky. *Nose* flat. *Lips* tumid. *Women* without shame. *Mammae* lactate profusely. *Crafty,* indolent, negligent. *Anoints* himself with grease. *Governed* by caprice'" (21; emphasis in original). When we choose to use shame, we are linking ourselves to these practices of operating within a shame-honor continuum, even if we find our own operations of use to be worthy. The deployment of shame is an act of communication that always relies on a hierarchy, a division between some righteousness and some unrighteousness.

Additionally, efforts to move past or release oneself from the binding effects of shame are also entirely understandable but worthy of ongoing consideration. Narratives that demonstrate a shamed person "breaking free from" or "releasing themselves" from shame abound. While I in no way wish to suggest that people experiencing shame are destined to remain in perpetually nonagentive states, this investigation of shame's endurance offers several important and related perspectives. First, shame can linger even when it might very reasonably seem to dissipate. In such instances, it is wise to examine how shame's rhetorical operations may be surreptitiously continuing, potentially in new and unrecognizable forms. Second, narratives of personal relationships to (i.e., transcendence beyond) shame are often just that: personal. Like other recovery scripts, they may be illuminating for their depiction of individual notions of transformation, but they very well may not prompt interrogation of shame's operations at structural levels. Further, personal redemption is a dangerous script when it recasts the ability to resist shame in ways that imply that doing so is a matter of personal will and fortitude. Finally, shame's "stickiness" is real, as I am reminded by one of the mothers I interviewed for this project. This mother has been in reunion with the son she gave up for adoption decades ago, but within the last few years the son has resisted communication, thus "closing" the door to an ongoing relationship. Sharing with me this news, she explains: "I still feel shame that I am 'rejected' again, even though rationally I understand it may have nothing to do with me, but with him." Shame's lasting effects can endure, seeping into emotional and sensorial cavities of our experience, even when we tell ourselves that they will not or should not.

What, then, if not using shame to fight shame or laboring to moving past it? I conclude by considering the recent writing of Chanel Miller, the woman who was raped by Stanford University student athlete Brock Turner in 2015 and whose anonymous victim impact statement has contributed significantly to recent conversations about surviving rape and contemporary rape culture. In her memoir, *Know My Name,* Miller (2019) reflects on how the feelings of shame related to having been raped are extraordinarily difficult to rupture. Before turning to Miller's own words, it is useful to call attention to how she might have been perceived and "heard," listened to and not listened to, as both the anonymous "Emily Doe" and then, later, as a memoirist. In her opinion piece in the *New York Times,* novelist Lisa Ko (2019) reflects on her (likely shared) assumption that Emily Doe was a white woman and her surprise, upon reading *Know My Name,* that Miller is Chinese American. Ko calls attention to Miller not being white because of the memoirist's simultaneous work to claim her identity, claim her voice, and claim her Chinese identity; Ko argues that by "naming herself," Miller "takes control of the narrative on her own terms and opens up more space for others who choose to do so." But in reflecting on her own default move to assume that Doe was white, Ko calls upon readers to recognize the many Asian American women who defy the "silent or submissive" stereotype as they speak out against sexual violence—naming Amanda Nguyen, Leah Lakshmi Piepzna-Samarasinha, Emma Sulowicz, and Connie Chung (among "many other survivors") as proof of her claim. So while I end by pointing to Miller's memoir as opening up a space not only for speaking up but also for reconsidering shame (if not necessarily breaking free from it, as Miller is often credited for having done), it is important to recognize how whiteness continues to operate—even if in subtextual and tacit ways—in relation to public understandings of women's sexual and reproductive lives, even when they are "listened to."

Reflecting on the emotional danger of reporting a rape, Miller (2019) refers to victims' social treatment as involving "being retraumatized, publicly shamed, psychologically tormented, and verbally mauled" (288). An act of alleged restitution riled up feelings of shame for Miller. She writes that at the end of Turner's incarceration (he served three months of a six-month conviction), she was in negotiation with Stanford University for potential payment for her therapy. Such an arrangement was possible if Miller promised not to bring litigation against the institution. Recalling her feelings about this deliberation, Miller admits that she primarily "feared the guilt and shame and stigma that arrives when any victim receives any sum of money" (299). In short, it was not only the shame of the rape that stayed with Miller in the months and years after the assault, but the various ways that shame emerged—or threatened to emerge—among wider publics as she moved forward with her healing and with her life.

Interestingly, Miller's recollection of a moment free of shame came as she was being examined by two nurses immediately after the assault, "I understood their gloved hands were keeping me from falling into an abyss. Whatever was crawling into the corridors of my insides would be dragged out by the ankles. They were a force, barricading me, even making me laugh. They could not undo what was done, but they could record it, photograph every millimeter of it, seal it into bags, force someone to look. Not once did they sigh or pity or *poor thing* me. They did not mistake my submission for weakness, so I did not feel a need to prove myself, to show them I was more than this. They knew. Shame could not breathe here" (13–14).

Although Miller's memoir could be classified as an example of writing shame, I am drawn to how Miller amplifies the feeling associated with a shame-free space—an embodied experience of existing outside of shame's reach. What might it mean for feminists to work coalitionally to not only account for shame, to not only write shame in ways that use sharing to name shame culture, but to proactively work to cultivate sites of sexual and reproductive knowledge-making that are truly free of shame? As feminist scholars continue to recover histories of reproduction and do activist work that seeks reproductive justice for all people, we must share, listen, and love toward building rhetorical practices and cultivating affective ecologies where shame cannot endure, cannot breathe.

Notes

Introduction: Sex, Shame, and Rhetoric

1. Not the real name of this interviewee. Throughout the book I have honored interviewees' preferences for being referred to by name or anonymized by a pseudonym.

2. Hiding and surrender were also practiced in Canada, Australia, and Spain (Rather 2012). The related but distinct practices of Ireland's Magdalen Laundries (Smith 2007) are another shocking example of women being punished for "their" sexual transgression.

Chapter 1: Unwed Pregnancy and Radial Rhetorics of Shame

1. According to Ann Fessler (2007, 8), 1.5 million women went away and surrendered a child between 1945 and 1973; another estimate is approximately 6 million women (Wilson-Buterbaugh n.d.). Wilson-Buterbaugh (2017) further discusses complications in accounting for these unknowable figures (36).

2. The term *erased* is also used in contemporary feminist writing that does not account for its potential violence (see Roy and Thompson 2019).

3. Wilson-Buterbaugh (2017) refers to such surrender as "the ubiquitous, fraudulent, unethical and coercive practices of churches, maternity home administrators, adoption caseworkers, and the public social welfare system" (19).

4. I use *memoried* to emphasize that memory actively shapes this interview "data," which I consider to add rhetorical richness to rather than detract from the "validity" of experiences that historically were systematically silenced.

5. Such misogyny aligns with Puritan and Victorian notions of women's morality being measured by their sexual purity (Bordo 2003, 117) but has much deeper roots. Jewish sage Ben Sira (180 B.C.E.) asserts that daughters unable to control their own sexuality could cause more damage to a father's honor than any other relation (Balla 2011, 54–55). The belief that an unchaste daughter brings shame upon the family has since come to represent transhemispheric *doxa* (Lerner 1986, 140; Leverenz 2012, 60).

6. Various publications of the Florence Crittenton Association demonstrate how façades of such homes represented unwed pregnancy within the community. Pictures of the houses—not residents—are prominent in organizational materials, such as brochures, annual reports, and the 1897 *Fourteen Years' Work among Erring Girls*.

7. Two interviewees explained that they felt adoption ultimately was the best option for them at the time of their pregnancy. These two women did not speak of the trauma of the relinquishment of their child as other interviewees did. However, the decision to surrender their children for adoption was the "best" choice for these women in large part because of the complications they expected to face as single, unwed mothers if they kept

their babies. (And, indeed, if they were actually permitted to keep their babies, since any discussion of mothers' rights were infrequent and usually not upheld.) Thus, although these women embraced the decision to relinquish more fully than other mothers I interviewed, I would not characterize the decision as one made free from the constraints explored in this chapter.

Chapter 2: New Permissiveness, Stigma, and Unwed Pregnancy in the Early 1970s

1. The Student Nonviolent Coordinating Committee (SNCC) earlier created and distributed "Genocide in Mississippi," a pamphlet opposing efforts by Mississippi state legislator David H. Glass in 1958 to enforce sterilization of mothers receiving welfare benefits. The legislation, focused on unwed mothers, was billed as a response to these women's "immorality." It passed overwhelmingly in the Mississippi State House but the not the Senate, thanks to SNCC protest (Washington 2008, 203; Roberts 2017, 94).

Chapter 3: Macrochange, Reproductive Agency, and the Stickiness of Shame

1. I thank Barbara Heifferon for suggesting this metaphor to me.

2. Many feminist/womanist scholars have written about this aspect of Sanger's legacy. See Davis 1983; Gordon 1994; López 2008; Roberts, 2017; and Schoen 2005.

3. See Adams 2019.

Chapter 4: Rhetorical Blame and Pregnant Teens in the Late 1970s

1. The popularity of the phrase "babies having babies" in the 1980s is suggested by several artistic productions. In 1986, Martin Sheen directed a "CBS Schoolbreak Special" that adapted Jeffrey Auerbach and Kathryn Montgomery's published play "Babies Having Babies" (Margulies 1986). Additionally, in 1988, R&B artist Terry Tate released the single "Babies Having Babies."

2. I use the term *adversity* to reflect struggle that is experienced and not to place judgment. I borrow this usage from compelling advocacy writing produced by National Crittenton, the current iteration of the Florence Crittenton Mission that I discuss more fully in the conclusion.

3. For a discussion of neoliberalism's slow violence, see Roy and Thompson 2019, 4–8.

4. The Institute of Society, Ethics and Life Sciences was a bioethics research center that would later become the Hastings Center.

5. An example of female-specific data is suggested by a chart that measures the "percent of births to females aged 14–19 that were out-of-wedlock, by single years of age, United States, 1960–1964–1970–1974" (14). An example of data that include males is "sources of contraception among sexually active teenagers, United States, 1971," which would presumably include males and females (43). These visuals are not reprints, but are representations of data gathered by AGI.

6. A *Nation* article offers a rare example of a moment of normalizing discourse in relation to teens and the teen pregnancy situation. The article argues that "teen sexual irresponsibility reflects the sexual discomfort and frustration felt by most adults, 50 percent of whom are sexually ignorant and/or unsatisfied, according to an estimate by the sex research team of Masters and Johnson" (Castleman 1977, 552). This bridge between teen activities/knowledges and adult activities/knowledges is uncommon in other articles, which depict teens as representing a wholly unique identity category.

7. Many of the articles quote individuals with an avowed knowledge of pregnant teenagers, such as psychologists, physicians, workers in teen pregnancy centers, researchers,

and so on. I use the term *expert* here in relation to how the articles solicit "expert" testimony from these individuals.

8. By counting raced bodies in the brochure and noticing a similar representation of whiteness in the magazines, I cautiously participate in a fiction of visible race difference.

9. My count is based on females who are seemingly the subject of the picture (e.g., they appear in the foreground and not in the background). A similar count of males in the brochure shows four males total: three males appear to be white and one male appears to be African American.

Conclusion: The Legacies of Righteous Reproduction

1. See Mann's (2018) discussion of unbounded shame that has no logical end other than self-destruction.

2. Hobbs sent a letter to parents of 9th through 12th-grade students to alert them that, in the words of Maddi's mother, "something had come up" (Wright and Hawkins 2017).

3. See Students for Life of America 2017, "Congrats."

Bibliography

"82 Sterilized by Alabama." *Washington Daily News,* July 1, 1973, n.p.

Adams, Heather Brook. "Goodbye, 'Post-Pill Paradise': Texturing Feminist Public Memories of Women's Reproductive and Rhetorical Agency." *Quarterly Journal of Speech* 105, no. 4 (2019): 390–417.

Adams, Mary Louise. *The Trouble with Normal: Postwar Youth and the Making of Heterosexuality.* Toronto: University of Toronto Press, 1997.

Adolescent Health Services, and Pregnancy Prevention Care Act of 1978: Hearing before the H. Subcomm. on Health and the Environment of the Committee on Interstate and Foreign Commerce, 95th Cong. (1978).

Adolescent Health Services, and Pregnancy Prevention Care Act of 1978: Hearing before the S. Subcomm. on Human Resources, 95th Cong. (1978).

Adolescent Pregnancy: Hearing before the H. Subcomm. on Select Education of the Committee on Education and Labor, 95th Cong. (1978).

Agnew, Lois, Laurie Gries, and Zosha Stuckey. "Introduction: Octalog III: The Politics of Historiography in 2010." *Rhetoric Review* 30, no. 2 (2011): 109–10.

Ahmed, Sara. *The Cultural Politics of Emotion.* New York: Routledge, 2004.

———. *The Promise of Happiness.* Durham, NC: Duke University Press, 2010.

Alan Guttmacher Institute. *11 Million Teenagers: What Can Be Done About the Epidemic of Adolescent Pregnancies in the United States.* New York: Author, 1976.

Allyn, David. *Make Love, Not War: The Sexual Revolution: An Unfettered History.* London: Routledge, 2001.

"Aunt Martha's Decline." *Newsweek,* March 27, 1972, 100.

Avery, Byllye Y. "Byllye Y. Avery." By Loretta Ross. Voices of Feminism Oral History Project. Southampton, MA: Smith College, 2005.

Balkin, Jack M., ed. *What* Roe v. Wade *Should Have Said: The Nation's Top Legal Experts Rewrite America's Most Controversial Decision.* New York: New York Univeristy Press, 2005.

Balla, Ibolya. *Ben Sira on Family, Gender, and Sexuality.* Berlin: Hubert, 2011.

Bartky, Sandra Lee. *Femininity and Domination.* New York: Routledge, 1990.

Bazelon, Emily, John Dickerson, and David Plotz. "The 'Live from Chicago' Edition." *Slate's Political Gabfest.* Slate.com, podcast audio, October 26, 2017.

Bellafante, Ginia. "Fantasies of Women, When They Were New." *New York Times,* February 24, 2007, B13.

Bernstein, Robin. *Racial Innocence: Performing American Childhood from Slavery to Civil Rights.* New York: New York University Press, 2011.

Bordo, Susan. *Unbearable Weight: Feminism, Western Culture, and the Body.* 10th anniversary edition. Berkeley: University of California Press, 2003.

Borelli, P. "The Real McCoys (1960)." *Television's New Frontier: The 1960s* (blog). February 15, 2012. tvnewfrontier.blogspot.com/search?q=the+real+mccoys.

Boston Women's Health Book Collective. *Our Bodies, Ourselves.* New York: Simon & Schuster, 1973.

Bower, Anne. "Bill Baird: The 30 Year Crusade." *Body Politic* 6, no. 2 (1996): 10.

Brake, Deborah L. *Getting in the Game: Title IX and the Women's Sports Revolution.* New York: New York University Press, 2010.

Brandt, Allan M. *No Magic Bullet: A Social History of Venereal Disease in the United States since 1880.* New York: Oxford University Press, 1985.

Brandzel, Amy L. *Against Citizenship: The Violence of the Normative.* Urbana: University of Illinois Press, 2016.

Brief for Appellant (New York Supreme Court, Appellate Division). June 22, 1917. *The Margaret Sanger Papers: Smith College Collections and Collected Documents Series,* Smith College, Northampton.

Briggs, Laura. *How All Politics Became Reproductive Politics: From Welfare Reform to Foreclosure to Trump.* Oakland: University of California Press, 2017.

———. *Reproducing Empire: Race, Sex, Science, and U.S. Imperialism in Puerto Rico.* Berkeley: University of California Press, 2003.

brown, adrienne maree. *We Will Not Cancel Us: And Other Dreams of Transformative Justice.* Chico, CA: AR Press, 2020.

Brown, Helen Gurley. *Sex and the Single Girl.* New York: Open Road Media, 2012. First published 1962.

Buchanan, Lindal. *Rhetorics of Motherhood.* Carbondale: Southern Illinois University Press, 2013.

Burke, Kenneth. *A Grammar of Motives.* Berkeley: University of California Press, 1962.

———. *Language as Symbolic Action.* Berkeley: University of California Press, 1968.

———. *Permanence and Change: An Anatomy of Purpose.* 3rd ed. Berkeley: University of California Press, 1965.

———. *The Philosophy of Literary Form.* 3rd ed. Berkeley: University of California Press, 1974.

Burke, Tarana, and Brené Brown, eds. *You Are Your Best Thing: Vulnerability, Shame Resilience, and the Black Experience.* New York: Random House, 2021.

Cade, Toni "The Pill: Genocide or Liberation?" In *The Black Woman: An Anthology,* edited by Toni Cade Bambara, New York: Washington Square Press, 1970.

Campbell, Karlyn Kohrs. "Agency: Promiscuous and Protean." *Communication and Critical/Cultural Studies* 2, no. 1 (2005): 1–19.

Cannon, Lou. *President Reagan: The Role of a Lifetime.* New York: Perseus, 2000.

Caron, Simone M. "Birth Control and the Black Community in the 1960s: Genocide or Power Politics?" *Journal of Social History* 31, no. 3 (1998): 545–69.

———. *Who Chooses? American Reproductive History since 1830.* Gainesville: University Press of Florida, 2008.

Carter, C. Allen. *Kenneth Burke and the Scapegoat Process.* Norman: University of Oklahoma Press, 1996.

Carter, Jimmy. "Inaugural Address." Washington, DC, January 20, 1977.

Castleman, Michael. "Why Teenagers Get Pregnant." *Nation,* November 26, 1977, 549–52.

Cedillo, Christina V., Victor Del Hierro, Candace Epps-Robertson, Lisa Michelle King, Jessie Male, Staci Perryman-Clark, Andrea Riley-Mukavetz, and Amy Vidali. "Listening to Stories: Practicing Cultural Rhetorics Pedagogy." *constellations: A Cultural Rhetorics*

Publishing Space 1. May 1, 2018. http://constell8cr.com/issue-1/listening-to-stories-practicing-cultural-rhetorics-pedagogy/.

Chappell, Marisa. *The War on Welfare: Family, Poverty, and Politics in Modern America.* Philadelphia: University of Pennsylvania Press, 2010.

Charmallas, Martha. "Unpacking Emotional Distress: Sexual Exploitation, Reproductive Harm, and Fundamental Rights." *Wake Forest Law Review* 44, no. 5 (2009): 1109–30.

Chase, Elaine, and Grace Bantebya-Kyomuhendo. Introduction. In *Poverty and Shame: Global Experiences,* edited by Elaine Chase and Grace Bantebya-Kyomuhendo, 1–20. Oxford, England: Oxford University Press, 2015.

Chávez, Karma R. "The Body: An Abstract and Actual Rhetorical Concept." *Rhetoric Society Quarterly* 48, no. 3 (2018): 242–50.

Chen, Jim. "Midnight in the Courtroom of Good and Evil." *Constitutional Commentary* 16, (1999): 499–504.

Cherlin, Andrew. "Carter Half Sees the Problem." *Nation,* June 17, 1978, 727–30.

Cherney, James L. "The Rhetoric of Ableism." *Disability Studies Quarterly* 31, no. 3 (2011).

Clow, Barbara. "'An Illness of Nine Months' Duration': Pregnancy and Thalidomide Use in Canada and the United States." In *Women, Health, and Nation: Canada and the United States since 1945,* edited by Georgina Feldberg, Molly Ladd-Taylor, Alison Li, and Kathryn McPherson, 45–66. Montreal: McGill-Queen's University Press, 2003.

Collins, Patricia Hill. *Black Feminist Thought: Knowledge, Consciousness, and the Politics of Empowerment.* 2nd ed. New York: Routledge, 2000.

Condit, Celeste Michelle. *Decoding Abortion Rhetoric: Communicating Social Change.* Urbana: University of Illinois Press, 1990.

Cook, Katsi. "Katsi Cook." By Joyce Follett. Voices of Feminism Oral History Project. Southampton, MA: Smith College, 2005.

———. "The Women's Dance." In *New Voices from the Longhouse: An Anthology of Contemporary Iroquois Writing,* edited by Joseph Bruchac, 80–89. Greenfield Center, NY: Greenfield Review Press, 1989.

Cushman, Ellen. "Translingual and Decolonial Approaches to Meaning Making." *College English* 78, no. 3 (2016): 234–42.

Dailey, Jane. *White Fright: The Sexual Panic at the Heart of America's Racist History.* New York: Basic Books, 2020.

Darity, W. A., and C. B. Turner. "Family Planning, Race Consciousness, and the Fear of Race Genocide." *American Journal of Public Health* 62, no. 11 (1972): 1454–59.

David, Marlo D. *Mama's Gun: Black Maternal Figures and the Politics of Transgression.* Columbus: Ohio State University Press, 2016.

Davis, Angela Y. *Women, Race, and Class.* New York: Vintage, 1983.

Demo, Anne Teresa. "Introduction: Reframing Motherhood: Factoring in Consumption and Privilege." In *The Motherhood Business: Consumption, Communication, and Privilege,* edited by Anne Teresa Demo, Jennifer L. Borda, and Charlotte Kr; 1–27. Tuscaloosa: University of Alabama Press, 2015.

Deonna, Julien A., Raffaele Rodogno, and Fabrice Teroni. *In Defense of Shame: The Faces of an Emotion.* New York: Oxford University Press, 2012.

Deparle, Jason, and Sabrina Tavernise. "Unwed Mothers Now a Majority before Age of 30." *New York Times,* February 18, 2012, 1+.

Department of Education. *Open to All: Title IX at Thirty.* 2003. https://www2.ed.gov/about/bdscomm/list/athletics/title9report.pdf.

de Souza, Rebecca. *Feeding the Other: Whiteness, Privilege, and Neoliberal Stigma in Food Pantries.* Cambridge, MA: MIT Press, 2019.

DiCaglio, Sara, and Lori Beth De Hertogh. "Introduction to "Rhetorical Pasts, Rhetorical Futures: Reflecting on the Legacy of *Our Bodies, Ourselves* and the Future of Feminist Health Literacy." *Peitho* 21, no. 3 (2019): 565–75.

Dolezal, Luna. *The Body and Shame: Phenomenology, Feminism, and the Socially Shaped Body.* Reprint, Lanham, MD: Lexington Books, 2016.

Dolmage, Jay Timothy. *Disability Rhetoric.* Syracuse, NY: Syracuse University Press, 2014.

Dolmage, Jay and Cynthia Lewiecki-Wilson. "Refiguring Rhetorica: Linking Feminist Rhetoric and Disability Studies." In *Rhetorica in Motion: Feminist Rhetorical Methods and Methodologies*, edited by Eileen E. Schell and K. J. Rawson, 23–38. Pittsburgh, PA: University of Pittsburgh Press, 2010.

Douglas, Mary. *Purity and Danger: An Analysis of Concept of Pollution and Taboo.* London: Routledge, 1966.

Draper, Allison. "The History of the Term Pudendum: Opening the Discussion on Anatomical Sex Inequality." *Clinical Anatomy* 34, no. 2 (2021): 315–19.

Dudley-Shotwell, Hannah. *Revolutionizing Women's Healthcare: The Feminist Self-Help Movement in America.* New Brunswick, NJ: Rutgers University Press, 2020.

Duncan, Nancy. "Renegotiating Gender and Sexuality in Public and Private Spaces." In *BodySpace: Destabilizing Geographies of Gender and Sexuality*, edited by Nancy Duncan, 127–44. London: Routledge, 1996.

Echols, Alice. *Daring to Be Bad: Radical Feminism in America 1967–1975.* Minneapolis: University of Minnesota Press, 1989.

Edin, Kathryn, and Maria Kefalas. *Promises I Can Keep: Why Poor Women Put Motherhood Before Marriage.* Berkeley: University of California Press, 2005.

Eisenstadt v. Baird. 405 US 438 (1972).

Elman, Julie Passanante. "After School Special Education: Rehabilitative Television, Teen Citizenship, and Compulsory Able-Bodiedness." *Television New Media* 11, no. 4 (2010): 260–92.

Enoch, Jessica. *Domestic Occupations: Spatial Rhetorics and Women's Work.* Carbondale: Southern Illinois University Press, 2019.

———. "Releasing Hold: Feminist Historiography without the Tradition." In *Theorizing Histories of Rhetoric*, edited by Michelle Baliff, 58–73. Carbondale: Southern Illinois University Press, 2013.

———. "Survival Stories: Feminist Historiographic Approaches to Chicana Rhetorics of Sterilization Abuse." *Rhetoric Society Quarterly* 35, no. 3 (2005): 5–30.

Epps-Robertson, Candace. *Resisting Brown: Race, Literacy, and Citizenship in the Heart of Virginia.* Pittsburgh, PA: University of Pittsburgh Press, 2018.

Erikson, Erik H. *Identity: Youth and Crisis.* New York: Norton, 1968.

Federici, Silvia. *Caliban and the Witch: Women, the Body and Primitive Accumulation.* New York: Autonomedia, 2014.

Fessler, Ann. *The Girls Who Went Away: The Hidden History of Women Who Surrendered Children for Adoption in the Decades Before Roe. v. Wade.* New York: Penguin, 2007.

Fields, Tanya Denise. "Dirty Business: The Messy Affair of Rejecting Shame." In *You Are Your Best Thing: Vulnerability, Shame Resilience, and the Black Experience*, edited by Tarana Burke and Brené Brown, 22–32. New York: Random House, 2021.

Fischer, Clara. "Gender and the Politics of Shame: A Twenty-First-Century Feminist Shame Theory." *Hypatia* 33, no. 3 (2018): 371–83.

Fixmer-Oraiz, Natalie. *Homeland Maternity: US Security Culture and the New Reproductive Regime.* Chicago: University of Illinois Press, 2019.

——. "No Exception Postprevention: 'Differential Biopolitics' on the Morning After." In *Contemplating Maternity in an Era of Choice: Explorations into Discourses of Reproduction,* edited by Sara Hayden and D. Lynn O'Brien Hallstein, 27–48. Lanham, MD: Lexington Books, 2010.

Flietz, Elizabeth. "Material." *Peitho Journal* 18, no. 1 (2015): 34–38.

Flippen, J. Brooks. *Jimmy Carter, the Politics of the Family, and the Rise of the Religious Right.* Athens: University of Georgia Press, 2011.

"Florence Crittenton Mission." VCU Libraries Social Welfare History Project, accessed March 15, 2019. socialwelfare.library.vcu.edu/programs/child-welfarechild-labor/florence-crittenton-mission/.

Fox, Margalit. "Barbara Seaman, 72, Dies; Cited Risks of the Pill." *New York Times,* March 1, 2008. https://www.nytimes.com/2008/03/01/nyregion/01seaman.html.

Fraser, Nancy, and Linda Gordon. "A Genealogy of 'Dependency': Tracing a Keyword of the U.S. Welfare State." In *Justice Interruptus: Critical Reflections on the "Postsocialist" Condition,* edited by Nancy Fraser, 121–49. New York: Routledge, 1997.

Freedman, Estelle B. *No Turning Back: The History of Feminism and the Future of Women.* New York: Ballantine, 2002.

Friday, Nancy. *My Secret Garden: Women's Sexual Fantasies.* New York: Pocket, 1973.

Fried, Malene Gerber. "Reproductive Rights Activism after *Roe.*" In *Radical Reproductive Justice: Foundations, Theory, Practice, Critique,* edited by Loretta J. Ross, Lynn Roberts, Erika Derkas, Whitney Peoples, and Pamela Bridgewater Toure, 139–50. New York: Feminist Press, 2017.

Frischherz, Michaela. "Affective Agency and Transformative Shame: The Voices Behind *The Great Wall of Vagina.*" *Women's Studies in Communication* 38 (2015): 251–72.

Furstenberg, Frank F. *Destinies of the Disadvantaged: The Politics of Teen Childbearing.* New York: Russel Sage Foundation, 2010.

Gallagher, Ursula M. "National Trends in Services to Unmarried Parents." Speech, Citizens Conference on Services to Unmarried Parents, Kansas City, MO, November 27, 1967. Transcript. Federal Government Social Welfare Publications. Department of Health, Education, and Welfare: Social and Rehabilitation Service: Children's Bureau, 1959–1969. Box 17. Social Welfare History Archive, University of Minnesota Library.

——. "What of the Unmarried Mother?" *Journal of Home Economics* 55, no. 6 (1963): 401–405.

Garland-Thomson, Rosemarie. "Integrating Disability, Transforming Feminist Theory." In *Feminist Disability Studies,* edited by Kim Q. Hall, 13–47. Bloomington: Indiana University Press, 2011.

——. "The Politics of Staring: Visual Representations of Disabled People in Popular Culture." *Disability Studies: Enabling the Humanities,* edited by Sharon L. Snyder, Brenda Jo Brueggemann, and Rosemarie Garland-Thomson, 56–75. New York: Modern Language Association, 2002.

Gibbs, Nancy. "Love, Sex, Freedom and the Paradox of the Pill." *Newsweek,* May 3, 2010, 40–47.

Gibson, Katie L. "The Rhetoric of *Roe v. Wade:* When the (Male) Doctor Knows Best." *Southern Communication Journal* 73, no. 4 (2008): 312–31.

Gilens, Martin. "How the Poor Became Black: The Racialization of American Poverty in the Mass Media." In *Race and the Politics of Welfare Reform,* edited by Sanford F. Schram, Joe Soss, and Richard C. Fording, 101–30. Ann Arbor: University of Michigan Press, 2003.

Glasser, Gabrielle. *American Baby: A Mother, a Child, and the Shadow History of Adoption.* New York: Viking, 2020.

Glenn, Cheryl. *Rhetoric Retold: Regendering the Tradition from Antiquity through the Renaissance.* Carbondale: Southern Illinois University Press, 1997.

——. *Rhetorical Feminism and This Thing Called Hope.* Carbondale: Southern Illinois University Press, 2018.

——. *Unspoken: A Rhetoric of Silence.* Carbondale: Southern Illinois University Press, 2004.

Goffman, Erving. *Stigma: Notes on the Management of Spoiled Identity.* New York: Simon & Schuster, 1963.

Gordon, Linda. *Pitied but Not Entitled: Single Mothers and the History of Welfare.* Detroit: Free Press, 1994.

Greenhouse, Linda. *Becoming Justice Blackmun: Harry Blackmun's Supreme Court Journey.* New York: Times Books, 2005.

Griswold v. State of Connecticut, 381 U.S. 479 (1965).

Guide Book for Our Home. n.d. Florence Crittenton Collection: NCFM Member Homes: Ohio. Box 23, Folder 5. Social Welfare History Archive, University of Minnesota Library.

Hall, Meredith. *Without a Map: A Memoir.* Boston: Beacon, 2007.

Hallenbeck, Sarah. *Claiming the Bicycle: Women, Rhetoric, and Technology in Nineteenth Century America.* Carbondale: Southern Illinois University Press, 2015.

Halliday, Aria S. "Introduction: Starting from Somewhere: Groundwork and Themes." In *The Black Girlhood Studies Collection,* edited by Aria S. Halliday, 1–20. Toronto: Canadian Scholars, 2019.

Halliwell, Martin. *American Culture in the 1950s.* Edinburgh: Edinburgh University Press, 2007.

Hammers, Michele L. "Talking About 'Down There': The Politics of Publicizing the Female Body through *The Vagina Monologues.*" *Women's Studies in Communication* 29, no. 2 (2006): 220–43.

Hancock, Ange-Marie. *The Politics of Disgust: The Public Identity of the Welfare Queen.* New York: New York University Press, 2004.

Harris-Perry, Melissa V. *Sister Citizen: Shame, Stereotypes, and Black Women in America.* New Haven, CT: Yale University Press, 2011.

Hartman, Saidiya. *Wayward Lives, Beautiful Experiments: Intimate Histories of Social Upheaval.* New York: W. W. Norton, 2019.

Hauser, Gerard A. "Aristotle on Epideictic: The Formation of Public Morality." *Rhetoric Society Quarterly* 29, no. 1 (1999): 5–23.

Hawn, Patti. *Good Girls Don't: A Memoir.* Scotts Valley, CA: Create Space, 2010.

Heim, Joe. "Christian School: Teen Banned from Graduation 'Not Because She Is Pregnant but Because She Was Immoral.'" *Washington Post,* May 24, 2017.

Hlavacik, Mark. *Assigning Blame: The Rhetoric of Education Reform.* Cambridge, MA: Harvard Education Press, 2016.

Hogeland, Lisa Maria. *Feminisms and Its Fictions: The Consciousness-Raising Novel and the Women's Liberation Movement.* Philadelphia: University of Pennsylvania Press, 1998.

Hogg, Charlotte. "Sorority Rhetorics as Everyday Epideictic." *College English* 80, no. 5 (2018): 423–48.

Hollander, John. "Honor Dishonorable: Shameful Shame." *Social Research* 70, no. 4 (2003): 1061–74.

Holloway, Karla FC. *Private Bodies, Public Texts: Race, Gender, and a Cultural Bioethics.* Durham, NC: Duke University Press, 2011.

Hood, Jay. "Desire and Fantasy in Erica Jong's *Fear of Flying*." In *This Book Is an Action: Feminist Print Culture and Activist Aesthetics*, edited by Jaime Harker and Cecilia Konchar Farr, 149–62. Urbana: University of Illinois Press, 2016.

Howard, Marion. "Pregnant School-Age Girls." *Journal of School Health* 41, no. 7 (1971): 361–64.

Hull, N. E. H., and Peter Charles Hoffer. *Roe v. Wade: The Abortion Rights Controversy in American History*. 2nd ed. Lawrence: University Press of Kansas, 2010.

"Imagine Being in a World of Nowhere." n.d. Crittenton Center Development Office. Child Welfare League of America Records, Series 3, Box 106, Florence Crittenton Division Executive Roundtable Meetings 1977 Folder. Social Welfare History Archive, University of Minnesota Library.

Jackson, Rachel C. "Resisting Relocation: Placing Leadership on Decolonized Indigenous Landscapes." *College English* 79, no. 5 (2017): 495–511.

Johnson, Erica L. and Patricia Moran, eds. *The Female Face of Shame*. Bloomington: Indiana University Press, 2013.

Johnson, Jenell. "The Skeleton on the Couch: The Eagleton Affair, Rhetorical Disability, and the Stigma of Mental Illness." *Rhetoric Society Quarterly* 40, no. 5 (2010): 459–78.

Johnson, Nan. *Gender and Rhetorical Space in American Life, 1866–1910*. Carbondale: Southern Illinois University Press, 2002.

Jong, Erica. *Fear of Flying*. New York: Open Road Media, 2013. First published 1973.

Kachlik, David. "Changes of Anatomical Nomenclature Must Be Deliberate: The Female External Genitalia." *Clinical Anatomy* 34, no. 2 (2021): 320–23.

Kasun, Jacqueline. "Teenage Pregnancy: Epidemic or Statistical Hoax?" *USA Today*, July 1978, 31–33.

Kearney, Melissa Schettini, and Phillip B. Levine. "Why Is the Teen Birth Rate in the United States So High and Why Does It Matter?" NBER Working Paper Series, National Bureau of Economic Research, 2012.

Kelly, Casey Ryan. "Donald J. Trump and the Rhetoric of *Ressentiment*." *Quarterly Journal of Speech* 106, no. 1 (2019): 2–24.

Kirkendall, Lester A., and Helen M. Cox. "Starting a Sex Education Program," *Children*. July-August 1967. 136–40. Federal Government Social Welfare Publications. Department of Health, Education, and Welfare: Social and Rehabilitation Service: Children's Bureau, 1968. Box 17. Social Welfare History Archive, University of Minnesota Library.

Kline, Wendy. *Bodies of Knowledge: Sexuality, Reproduction, and Women's Health in the Second Wave*. Chicago: University of Chicago Press, 2010.

Kluchin, Rebecca M. *Fit to Be Tied: Sterilization and Reproductive Rights in America, 1950–1980*. New Brunswick, NJ: Rutgers University Press, 2009.

Ko, Lisa. "Why It Matters That 'Emily Doe' in the Brock Turner Case Is Asian-American." *New York Times*, September 24, 2019. https://www.nytimes.com/2019/09/24/opinion/chanel-miller-know-my-name.html.

Koerber, Amy. *From Hysteria to Hormones: A Rhetorical History*. University Park: Pennsylvania State University Press, 2018.

———. "From Hysteria to Hormones and Back Again: Centuries of Outrageous Remarks about Female Biology." *Rhetoric of Health and Medicine* 1, no. 1–2 (2018): 179–92.

Kovach, Bill. "Birth Law Upset in Massachusetts." *New York Times*, July 7, 1970. nytimes.com/1970/07/07/archives/birth-law-upset-in-massachusetts-us-court-rules-that-ban-on.html.

Lawrence, Jane. "The Indian Health Service and the Sterilization of Native American Women." *American Indian Quarterly* 24, no. 3 (2000): 400–19.

Le Guin, Ursula K. *Words Are My Matter: Writings About Life and Books 2000–2016.* Easthampton, MA: Small Beer Press, 2016.

Leonard, Toni M. Bond. "Laying the Foundations for a Reproductive Justice Movement." In *Radical Reproductive Justice: Foundations, Theory, Practice, Critique,* edited by Loretta J. Ross, Lynn Roberts, Erika Derkas, Whitney Peoples, and Pamela Bridgewater Toure, 39–49. New York: Feminist Press, 2017.

Lerner, Gerder. *The Creation of Patriarchy.* New York: Oxford University Press, 1986.

Leverenz, David. *Honor Bound: Race and Shame in America.* New Brunswick, NJ: Rutgers University Press, 2012.

Levine, Paul, and Harry Papasotiriou. *America since 1945: The American Moment.* New York: Red Globe, 2010.

Lincoln, Richard. "Is Pregnancy Good for Teenagers?" *USA Today,* July 1978, 34–37.

Link, Bruce G., and Jo C. Phelan. "Conceptualizing Stigma." *Annual Review of Sociology* 27, (2010): 363–85.

Locke, Jill. *Democracy and the Death of Shame: Political Equality and Social Disturbance.* New York: Cambridge University Press, 2016.

———. "Shame and the Future of Feminism." *Hypatia* 22, no. 4 (2007): 146–62.

López, Iris Ofelia. *Matters of Choice: Puerto Rican Women's Struggle for Reproductive Freedom.* New Brunswick, NJ: Rutgers University Press, 2008.

Lord, Alexandra M. *Condom Nation: The U.S. Government's Sex Education Campaign from World War I to the Internet.* Baltimore, MD: Johns Hopkins University Press, 2010.

Lucas, Roy. "New Historical Insights on the Curious Case of *Baird v Eisenstadt.*" *Roger Williams University Law Review* 9 (2003–2004): 9–55.

Luker, Kristin. *Abortion and the Politics of Motherhood.* Berkeley: University of California Press, 1984.

———. *Dubious Conceptions: The Politics of Teenage Pregnancy.* Cambridge, MA: Harvard University Press, 1997.

Lyerly, Anne Drapkin. "Shame, Gender, Birth." *Hypatia* 21, no. 1 (2006): 101–18.

Madrigal v. Quilligan, No. 75-2057, Ninth Circuit US District Court (1978).

Manion, Jennifer C. "Girls Blush, Sometimes: Gender, Moral Agency, and the Problem of Shame." *Hypatia* 18, no. 3 (2003): 21–41.

Mann, Bonnie. "Femininity, Shame, and Redemption." *Hypatia* 33, no. 3 (2018): 402–17.

Mannix von Zerneck, Julie, and Kathy Hatfield. *Secret Storms: A Mother and Daughter, Lost then Found.* Toluca Lake, CA: Blue Blazer, 2013.

Margulies, Lee. "TV Reviews: 'Melba' and 'Babies Having Babies.'" *Los Angeles Times,* January 28, 1986, 8.

Marks, Judy. "Teens and Pregnancy: No Easy Answers." *Teen,* September 1979, 24+.

Martinez, Aja Y. *Counterstory: The Rhetoric and Writing of Critical Race Theory.* Champaign, IL: National Council of Teachers of English, 2020.

Massumi, Brian. "The Future Birth of the Affective Fact: The Political Ontology of Threat." In *The Affect Theory Reader,* edited by Melissa Gregg and Gregory J. Seigworth, 52–70. Durham, NC: Duke University Press, 2010.

May, Elaine Tyler. *America and The Pill: A History of Promise, Peril, and Liberation.* New York: Basic-Perseus, 2010.

———. *Homeward Bound: American Families in the Cold War Era.* Rev. ed. New York: Basic-Perseus, 2008.

McConnell, Nancy Fifield, and Martha Morrison Dore. *1883–1983 Crittenton Services: The First Century.* Washington DC: National Florence Crittenton Mission, 1983.

McDowell, Linda. *Gender, Identity, and Place: Understanding Feminist Geographies.* Minneapolis: University of Minnesota Press, 1999.

McRuer, Robert. *Crip Theory: Cultural Signs of Queerness and Disability.* New York: New York University Press, 2006.

McWatt, Tessa. *Shame on Me: An Anatomy of Race and Belonging.* Toronto: Random House Canada, 2020.

Melcher, Mary S. *Pregnancy, Motherhood, and Choice in Twentieth-Century Arizona.* Tucson: University of Arizona Press, 2012.

Mendible, Myra. Introduction to *American Shame: Stigma and the Body Politic,* edited by Myra Mendible, 1–23. Bloomington: Indiana University Press, 2016.

Metalious, Grace. *Peyton Place.* Boston: Northeastern University Press. 1956.

Miller, Carolyn R. "What Can Automation Tell Us About Agency?" *Rhetoric Society Quarterly* 37, no. 2 (2007): 137–57.

Miller, Chanel. "I Am with You." Viking Books, September 24, 2019. YouTube video, 5:09, https://www.youtube.com/watch?v=0uIxvBMF7Rw.

——. *Know My Name: A Memoir.* New York: Viking, 2019.

Miller, Elisabeth. "Too Fat to be President?: Chris Christie and Fat Stigma as Rhetorical Disability." *Rhetoric of Health & Medicine* 2, no. 1 (2019): 60–87.

Mink, Patsy. "Statement by Representative Patsy T. Mink In the US House of Representatives Concerning Hyde Amendment on Abortion." August 1976. Patsy Mink Papers, Library of Congress.

Mittelstadt, Jennifer. "Educating 'Our Girls' and 'Welfare Mothers': Discussions of Education Policy for Pregnant and Parent Adolescents in Federal Hearings, 1975–1995." *Journal of Family History* 22, no. 3 (1997): 326–53.

Moorman, Margaret. *Waiting to Forget: A Motherhood Lost and Found.* New York: W.W. Norton, 1996.

Morgan, Robin. "Goodbye to All That." In *Dear Sisters: Dispatches from the Women's Liberation Movement,* edited by Rosalyn Baxandall and Linda Gordon, 53–57. New York: Basic Books, (1970) 2000.

Morrison, Joseph L. "Illegitimacy, Sterilization, and Racism: A North Carolina Case History." *Social Service Review* 39, no. 1 (1965): 1–10.

Moslener, Sara. *Virgin Nation: Sexual Purity and American Adolescence.* New York: Oxford University Press, 2015.

Mountford, Roxanne. *The Gendered Pulpit: Preaching in American Protestant Spaces.* Carbondale: Southern Illinois University Press, 2003.

Moynihan, Daniel Patrick. *The Moynihan Report: The Negro Family—The Case for National Action, 1965.* New York: Cosimo, 2018.

Murphy, John M. "Epideictic and Deliberative Strategies in Opposition to War: The Paradox of Honor and Expediency." *Communication Studies* 43, no. 2 (1992): 65–78.

Murray, Melissa. "The Space Between: The Cooperative Regulation of Criminal Law and Family Law." *Family Law Quarterly* 44, no. 2 (2010): 227.

"My Problem and How I Solved It: I Was Sixteen, Unmarried—and Expecting a Baby." *Good Housekeeping,* May 1980, 30+.

Naismith, Grace. "Teen-Age Sexuality: Too Many Pregnancies Too Early." *Reader's Digest,* November 1977, 150–52.

Nakkula, Michael J., and Eric Toshalis. *Understanding Youth: Adolescent Development for Educators.* Cambridge, MA: Harvard Education Press, 2006.

Nelson, Jennifer. *Women of Color and the Reproductive Rights Movement.* New York: New York University Press, 2003.

Newburger, Emma. "Trump Responds to E. Jean Carroll's Sexual Assault Accusations: 'Shame on Those Who Make up False Stories of Assault." *CNBC*, June 21, 2019.

Nicotra, Jodi. "Disgust, Distributed: Virtual Public Shaming as Epideictic Assemblage." *Enculturation* 6 (2016).

Nillson, Jeff, and Steven M. Spencer. "1965: The Birth Control Revolution." *Saturday Evening Post,* December 31, 2015. saturdayeveningpost.com/2015/12/50-years-ago-the-birth-control-revolution/.

Nunley, Vorris L. *Keepin' It Hushed: The Barbershop and African American Hush Harbor Rhetoric.* Detroit, MI: Wayne State University Press, 2011.

Nussbaum, Martha C. *Hiding from Humanity: Disgust, Shame, and the Law.* Princeton, NJ: Princeton University Press, 2004.

O'Hara, Mary. *The Shame Game: Overturning the Toxic Poverty Narrative.* Bristol, UK: Policy Press, 2020.

Okeowo, Alexis. "How Saidiya Hartman Retells the History of Black Life." *New Yorker,* October 26, 2020.

Ordover, Nancy. *American Eugenics: Race, Queer Anatomy, and the Science of Nationalism.* Minneapolis: University of Minnesota Press, 2003.

Ordway v. Hargraves, 323 F. Supp. 1155 (US D. Mass. 1971).

Owens, Deirdre Cooper. *Medical Bondage: Race, Gender, and the Origins of American Gynecology.* Athens: University of Georgia Press, 2017.

Panetta, Edward M., and Marouf Hasian, Jr. "Anti-Rhetoric as Rhetoric: The Law and Economics Movement." *Communication Quarterly* 42, no. 1 (1994): 57–74.

Parascandola, John. *Sex, Sin, and Science: A History of Syphilis in America.* Westport, CT: Praeger, 2008.

Parks, Suzan-Lori. *Getting Mother's Body.* New York: Random House, 2004.

Paul, Eve W., Harriet F. Pilpel, and Nancy F. Wechsler. "Pregnancy, Teenagers, and the Law, 1974." *Family Planning Perspectives* 6, no. 3 (1974): 142–47.

Pember, Mary Annette. "'Amá' and the Legacy of Sterilization in Indian Country." *Rewire News Group,* March 15, 2018. rewire.news/article/2018/03/15/ama-legacy-sterilization-indian-country/.

Perlman, Helen Harris. "Unmarried Mothers, Immorality, and the A.D.C." Annual Conference of the Florence Crittenton Association of America. Cleveland, Ohio. May 21, 1963. Transcript. Florence Crittenton Collection: FCAA Publications. Box 50, Folder 1. Social Welfare History Archive, University of Minnesota Library.

Perry v. Grenada Municipal Separate School District, 300 F Sup 748 (US D. Court N.D. Miss. 1969).

Phrydas, Irene. "Emotional Problems of the Unmarried Pregnant Girls and the Patterns of Denial Before and During Pregnancy." Southern Area Conference of the Florence Crittenton Association of America. Chattanooga. October 26, 1964. Transcript. Florence Crittenton Collection: FCAA Publications. Box 50, Folder 2. Social Welfare History Archive, University of Minnesota.

Pillow, Wanda S. *Unfit Subjects: Educational Policy and the Teen Mother.* New York: Routledge Falmer, 2004.

Posner, Richard A. *Sex and Reason.* Cambridge, MA: Harvard University Press, 1992.

Postman, Neil. *The Disappearance of Childhood.* New York: Vintage, 1994.

Powell, Malea. "2012 CCCC Chair's Address: Stories Take Place: A Performance in One Act." *College Composition and Communication* 64, no. 2 (2012): 383–406.

"Pregnant Teens." *Newsweek,* May 1977, 54.

Price, Kimala. "What is Reproductive Justice? How Women of Color Activists are Redefining the Pro-Choice Paradigm." *Meridians* 10, no. 2 (2010): 42–65.

Probyn, Elspeth. "Writing Shame." In *The Affect Theory Reader,* edited by Melissa Gregg and Gregory J. Seigworth, 71–90. Durham, NC: Duke University Press, 2010.

Rand, Erin J. "Bad Feelings in Public: Rhetoric, Affect, and Emotion." *Rhetoric and Public Affairs* 18, no. 1 (2015): 161–75.

———. *Reclaiming Queer: Activist and Academic Rhetorics of Resistance.* Tuscaloosa: University of Alabama Press, 2014.

Ratcliffe, Krista. *Rhetorical Listening: Identification, Gender, Whiteness.* Carbondale: Southern Illinois University Press, 2006.

———. "Silence and Listening: The War On/Over Women's Bodies in the 2012 US Election Cycle." In *Retellings: Opportunities for Feminist Research in Rhetoric and Composition Studies,* edited by Jessica Enoch and Jordynn Jack, 34–53. Anderson, SC: Parlor Press, 2019.

Rather, Dan. "Adopted or Abducted?" *Yahoo! News,* March 27, 2012. yahoo.com/news/forced-adoptions-for-unwed-mothers-around-the-globe.html.

Reagan, Leslie J. *When Abortion Was a Crime: Women, Medicine, and Law in the United States, 1867–1973.* Berkeley: University of California Press, 1998.

Rich, Adrienne. *On Lies, Secrets, and Silence: Selected Prose 1966–1978.* New York: W.W. Norton, 1979.

Rielly, Edward J. *The 1960s.* Santa Barbara, CA: Greenwood, 2003.

"Rising Concern over Surge in Illegitimacy." *U.S. News and World Report,* June 26, 1978, 59–60.

Robbins, Sarah. *Managing Literacy, Mothering America: Women's Narratives on Reading and Writing in the Nineteenth Century.* Pittsburgh, PA: University of Pittsburgh Press, 2004.

Roberts, Dorothy. *Killing the Black Body: Race, Reproduction, and the Meaning of Liberty.* 2nd ed. New York: Vintage, 2017.

Roberts, Lynn, Loretta Ross, and M. Bahati Kuumba. "The Reproductive Health and Sexual Rights of Women of Color: Still Building a Movement." *NWSA Journal* 17, no. 1 (2005): 93–98.

Roberts, Robert W. "A Theoretical Overview of the Unwed Mother." *The Unwed Mother,* 11–22. New York: Harper & Row, 1966.

Roe v. Wade, 410 S. Ct. 113 (1973).

Rogers, Annie G. *The Unsayable: The Hidden Language of Trauma.* New York: Random House, 2006.

Romano, Aja. "Why We Can't Stop Fighting about Cancel Culture." *Vox,* December 30, 2019. vox.com/culture/2019/12/30/20879720/what-is-cancel-culture-explained-history-debate.

Romano, Renee C., and Claire Bond Potter. "Just over Our Shoulder: The Pleasures and Perils of Writing the Recent Past." In *Doing Recent History: On Privacy, Copyright, Video Games, Institutional Review Boards, Activist Scholarship, and History That Talks Back,* edited by Claire Bond Potter and Renee C. Romano, 1–19. Athens: University of Georgia Press, 2012.

Ross, Loretta J. "Conceptualizing Reproductive Justice Theory: A Manifesto for Activism." In *Radical Reproductive Justice: Foundations, Theory, Practice, Critique,* edited by Loretta J. Ross, Lynn Roberts, Erika Derkas, Whitney Peoples, and Pamela Bridgewater Toure, 170–232. New York: Feminist Press, 2017.

——. "I'm a Black Feminist. I Think Call-Out Culture Is Toxic." *New York Times,* August 17, 2019. nyti.ms/2NcRJZG.

Ross, Loretta. "Loretta Ross." By Joyce Follett. Voices of Feminism Oral History Project, Southampton, MA: Smith College, 2004–2005.

Ross, Loretta J., Lynn Roberts, Erika Derkas, Whitney Peoples, and Pamela Bridgewater Toure. Introduction. In *Radical Reproductive Justice: Foundations, Theory, Practice, Critique,* edited by Loretta J. Ross, Lynn Roberts, Erika Derkas, Whitney Peoples, and Pamela Bridgewater Toure, 11–31. New York: Feminist Press, 2017.

Ross, Loretta J., and Rickie Solinger. *Reproductive Justice: An Introduction.* Oakland: University of California Press, 2017.

Rountree, Clarke. "The (Almost) Blameless Genre of Classical Greek Epideictic." *Rhetorica* 19, no. 3 (2001): 293–305.

Rowan, Carl T. "Judge Opens School Doors to Unwed Teen Mothers." *Spokane Daily Chronicle,* July 14, 1969, final fireside ed., sec. 1, 4.

Roy, Modhumita, and Mary Thompson, eds. *The Politics of Reproduction: Adoption, Abortion, and Surrogacy in the Age of Neoliberalism.* Columbus: Ohio State University Press, 2019.

Royster, Jacqueline Jones, and Gesa E. Kirsch. *Feminist Rhetorical Practices: New Horizons for Rhetoric, Composition, and Literacy Studies.* Carbondale: Southern Illinois University Press, 2012.

Runkles, Madeline. "I Got Pregnant. I Chose to Keep My Baby. And My Christian School Humiliated Me." *Chicago Tribune,* June 1, 2017. chicagotribune.com/opinion/commen tary/ct-pregnant-teen-christian-school-20170601-story.html.

"Salvation Army to Close Unwed Mothers Hospital." *San Diego Union,* December 17, 1971. Vertical File Collection: Women's Social Services Rescue Homes (Unwed Mothers). Alexandria, VA: Salvation Army Archives and Research Center.

Schaefer, Carol. *The Other Mother: A Woman's Love for the Child She Gave Up for Adoption.* New York: Soho, 1991.

Scheff, Thomas J. "Shame and the Social Bond: A Sociological Theory." *Sociological Theory* 18, no. 1 (2000): 84–99.

Schell, Eileen E. "Introduction: Researching Feminist Rhetorical Methods." In *Rhetorica in Motion: Feminist Rhetorical Methods and Methodologies,* edited by Eileen E. Schell and K. J. Rawson, 23–38. Pittsburgh, PA: University of Pittsburgh Press, 2010.

Schillinger, Liesl. "A Woman's Fantasy in a Modern Reality." *New York Times,* Dec. 20, 2013, p. E10. https://www.nytimes.com/2013/12/19/fashion/Fear-of-Flying-Erica-Jong .html.

Schoen, Johanna. *Choice and Coercion: Birth Control, Sterilization, and Abortion in Public Health and Welfare.* New ed. Chapel Hill: University of North Carolina Press, 2005.

Schuller, Kyla. *The Biopolitics of Feeling: Race, Sex, and Science in the Nineteenth Century.* Durham, NC: Duke University Press, 2018.

Schwartz, Tony. "Pregnant Teens." *Newsweek,* May 30, 1977, 54+.

Seaman, Barbara. *The Doctor's Case Against the Pill.* New York: Peter H. Wyden, 1969.

Segal, Judy Z. *Health and the Rhetoric of Medicine.* Carbondale: Southern Illinois University Press, 2005.

Seibers, Tobin. *Disability Theory.* Ann Arbor: University of Michigan Press, 2008.

Seigel, Marika. *The Rhetoric of Pregnancy.* Chicago: University of Chicago Press, 2014.

Shabot, Sara Cohen, and Keshet Korem. "Domesticating Bodies: The Role of Shame in Obstetric Violence." *Hypatia* 33, no. 3 (2018): 384–401.

Sharma, Sarah. "Baring Life and Lifestyle in the Non-Place." *Cultural Studies* 23, no. 1 (2009): 129–48.

Sharples, Madeline. "Introducing Patti Hawn, Author of *Good Girls Don't*." March 15, 2016. madelinesharples.com/tag/patti-hawn/.

Sheard, Cynthia Miecznikowski. "The Public Value of Epideictic Rhetoric." *College English* 58, no. 7 (1996): 765–94.

Shriver, Eunice Kennedy. "Teen-age Sexuality: There Is a Moral Dimension." *Reader's Digest,* November 1977, 153–4.

Siegel, J. A. "Letter." *Life,* April 23, 1971, 20A.

Silliman, Jael, Marlene Gerber Fried, Loretta Ross, and Elena R. Gutiérraez. *Undivided Rights: Women of Color Organize for Reproductive Justice.* Cambridge, MA: South End Press, 2004.

Slater, Jack. "The Growing Problem of Teen-Age Pregnancies." *Ebony,* March 1980, 53+.

Smith, James M. *Ireland's Magdalen Laundries and the Nation's Architecture of Containment.* Notre Dame, LA: University of Notre Dame Press, 2007.

Solinger, Rickie, "'A Complete Disaster': Abortion and the Politics of Hospital Abortion Committees, 1950–1970." *Feminist Studies* 19, no. 2 (1993): 240–68.

——. ed. *Abortion Wars: A Half Century of Struggle, 1950–2000.* Berkeley: University of California Press, 1998.

——. *Beggars and Choosers: How the Politics of Choice Shapes Adoption, Abortion, and Welfare in the United States.* New York: Hill and Wang, 2001.

——. *Pregnancy and Power: A Short History of Reproductive Politics in America.* New York: New York University Press, 2007.

——. *Wake Up Little Susie: Single Pregnancy and Race before* Roe v. Wade. New York: Routledge, 2000.

Spigel, Lynn. *Make Room for TV: Television and the Family Ideal in Postwar America.* Chicago: University of Chicago Press, 1992.

Spruill, Marjorie J. *Divided We Stand: The Battle Over Women's Rights and Family Values that Polarized American Politics.* London: Bloomsbury, 2017.

Stenberg, Shari J. "'Tweet Me Your First Assaults': Writing Shame and the Rhetorical Work of #NotOkay." *Rhetoric Society Quarterly* 48, no. 2 (2018): 119–138.

Stephens, Bret. "Trump and the Annihilation of Shame." *New York Times,* April 12, 2019. https://www.nytimes.com/2019/04/12/opinion/charles-van-doren-trump.html.

Stolberg, Sheryl Gay. "Pregnant at 18. Hailed by Abortion Foes. Punished by Christian School." *New York Times,* May 20, 2017. nytimes.com/2017/05/20/us/teen-pregnancy-religious-values-christian-school.html.

Stormer, Nathan. "Articulation: A Working Paper on Rhetoric and Taxis." *Quarterly Journal of Speech* 90, no. 3 (2004): 257–84.

Strickler, Rachael, and Monica Simpson. "A Brief Herstory of SisterSong." In *Radical Reproductive Justice: Foundations, Theory, Practice, Critique,* edited by Loretta J. Ross, Lynn Roberts, Erika Derkas, Whitney Peoples, and Pamela Bridgewater Toure, 50–57. New York: Feminist Press, 2017.

Students for Life of America, "About Us." Students for Life of America. 2017. studentsforlife.org/about/.

——. "Autumn's Response to Maddi: 'I Support You 100%.'" Students for Life of America, May 23, 2017. studentsforlife.org/2017/05/23/autumns-response-to-maddi-i-support-you-100/.

——. "Congrats to Maddi Runkles on Her High School Graduation!" Students for Life of

America, June 3, 2017. studentsforlife.org/2017/06/03/congrats-to-maddi-runkles-on
-her-high-school-graduation/.

———. "Martha MacCallum: Kristan Hawkins & Maddi Runkles." YouTube video, July 21,
2017. www.youtube.com/watch?v=k8ifNB1ctk8.

Sullivan, Dale L. "The Epideictic Rhetoric of Science." *Journal of Business and Technical
Communication* 5, no. 3 (1991): 229–45.

Tajima-Peña, Renee. Director. *No Más Bebés*. Latino Public Broadcasting, 2015.

Taylor, Dianna. "Humiliation as a Harm of Sexual Violence: Feminist versus Neoliberal
Perspectives." *Hypatia* 33, no. 3 (2018): 434–50.

"The Teenage Pregnancy Epidemic." *McCall's*, July 1978, 45–52.

"The Teen Pregnancy Problem: A New Approach." *Seventeen*, February 1980, 136+.

Theobald, Brianna. *Reproduction on the Reservation: Pregnancy, Childbirth, and Colonial-
ism in the Long Twentieth Centuries*. Chapel Hill: University of North Carolina Press,
2019.

There Is Time to Think. Florence Crittenton Collection: NCFM Member Homes: Philadelphia, PA. Box 23, Folder 12. Social Welfare History Archive, University of Minnesota
Library.

Thompson, M. Cordell. "Black Youngsters are Sterilized by Alabama Agency." *Jet*, July 19,
1973, 12–15.

Threadcraft, Shatema. *Intimate Justice: The Black Female Body and the Body Politic*. New
York: Oxford University Press, 2018.

Title IX, Education Amendments of 1972. Title 20 U.S.C. Sec. 1681–1688.

Torpy, Sally J. "Native American Women and Coerced Sterilization: On the Trail of Tears
in the 1970s." *American Indian Culture and Research Journal* 24, no. 2 (2000): 1–22.

Treichler, Paula A. *How to Have Theory in an Epidemic: Cultural Chronicles of AIDS*.
Durham, NC: Duke University Press, 1999.

Tuana, Nancy. "The Speculum of Ignorance: the Women's Health Movement and Epistemologies of Ignorance." *Hypatia* 21, no. 3 (2006): 1–19.

Tucker, Lorna. Director. *Amá*. London: Raindog Films, 2018. eVideo.

Turner C. B, and W. A. Darity. "Fears of Genocide among Black Americans as Related to
Age, Sex, and Religion." *American Journal of Public Health* 63, no. 12 (1973): 1029–34.

Valdes, Marcela. "When Doctors Took 'Family Planning' Into Their Own Hands." *New
York Times Magazine*, February 1, 2016. nytimes.com/2016/02/01/magazine/when
-doctors-took-family-planning-into-their-own-hands.html.

Valenti, Jessica. *The Purity Myth: How America's Obsession with Virginity Is Hurting Young
Women*. Berkeley, CA: Seal, 2009.

Vile, John R. *Essential Supreme Court Decisions: Summaries of Leading Cases in U.S. Constitutional Law*. 15th ed. Lanham, MD: Rowman & Littlefield, 2010.

Vinovskis, Maris A. *An "Epidemic" of Adolescent Pregnancy?: Some Historical and Policy
Considerations*. New York: Oxford University Press, 1988.

Vinson, Jenna. *Embodying the Problem: The Persuasive Power of the Teen Mother*. New
Brunswick, NJ: Rutgers University Press, 2018.

Warner, Michael. *The Trouble with Normal: Sex, Politics, and the Ethics of Queer Life*. New
ed. Cambridge, MA: Harvard University Press, 1999.

Washington, Harriet A. *Medical Apartheid: The Dark History of Medical Experimentation
on Black Americans from Colonial Times to the Present*. New York: Anchor, 2008.

Watkins, Elizabeth Siegel. *On the Pill: A Social History of Oral Contraceptives, 1950–1970*.
Baltimore, MD: Johns Hopkins University Press, 1998.

Watkins, Thomas H., Jr. "Sordid Sterilization." *Daily Challenge*, July 17, 1973, n.p.

Wax, Judith. "Teen Pregnancy: Whose Fault?" *Seventeen*, October 1978, 132+.

Weingarten, Karen. "Shame Before the Law: Affects of Abortion Regulation." In *American Shame: Stigma and the Body Politic*, edited by Myra Mendible, 27–43. Bloomington: Indiana University Press, 2016.

Weiss, Kay. "What Medical Students Learn about Women." In *Seizing Our Bodies: The Politics of Women's Health*, edited by Claudia Dreifus. New York: Vintage, 1977.

Welch, Nancy. "Ain't Nobody's Business: A Public Personal History of Privacy after *Baird v. Eisenstadt*." In *The Private, the Public, and the Published: Reconciling Private Lives and Public Rhetoric*, edited by Barbara Couture and Thomas Kent, 17–30. Logan: Utah State University Press, 2004.

Wells, Susan. *Our Bodies, Ourselves and the Work of Writing*. Stanford, CA: Stanford University Press, 2010.

Welter, Barbara. "The Cult of True Womanhood: 1820–1860." *American Quarterly* 18, no. 2 (1966): 151–74.

Wilson-Buterbaugh, Karen. *The Baby Scoop Era: Unwed Mothers, Infant Adoption and Forced Surrender*. Author, 2017.

——. "Setting the Record Straight." *Moxie Magazine*, moxiemag.com/moxie/articles/perspectives2.html.

Winderman, Emily. "Anger's Volumes: Rhetorics of Amplification and Aggregation in #MeToo." *Women's Studies in Communication* 42, no. 3 (2019): 327–46.

——. "S(anger) Goes Postal in *The Woman Rebel*: Angry Rhetoric as a Collectivizing Moral Emotion." *Rhetoric and Public Affairs* 17, no. 3 (2014): 381–420.

Wolf, Jacqueline H. *Deliver Me from Pain: Anesthesia and Birth in America*. Baltimore:, MD John Hopkins University Press, 2009.

Woodbury, Richard. "Help for High School Mothers." *Life*, April 2, 1971, 34–41.

Woodward, Kenneth L. "Saving the Family." *Newsweek*, May 15, 1978, 63+.

Wright, David, and Sally Hawkins. "A Pregnant Teen in a Class by Herself." *ABC News*, June 30, 2017. abcnews.go.com/US/pregnant-teen-class/story?id=48361156.

Wright, Elizabethada A. "'The Caprices of an Undisciplined Fancy': Using Blame to Negotiate the 'betweens' of *Ethos* via Epideictic." *Rhetoric Review* 38, no. 3 (2019): 271–84.

Yam, Shui-yin Sharon. "Visualizing Birth Stories from the Margin: Toward a Reproductive Justice Model of Rhetorical Analysis." *Rhetoric Society Quarterly* 50, no. 1 (2020): 19–34.

Yoder, Katie. "NBC, Fox Shed Light on Viral Story of 'Brave' Pregnant Teen Maddi Runkles." *News Busters*, May 26, 2017. www.newsbusters.org/blogs/culture/katie-yoder/2017/05/26/nbc-fox-shed-light-viral-story-brave-pregnant-teen-maddi.

Young, Isis Marion. *On Female Body Experience: Throwing Like a Girl and Other Essays*. New York: Oxford University Press, 2005.

Zavella, Patricia. *The Movement for Reproductive Justice: Empowering Women of Color through Social Activism*. New York: New York University Press, 2020.

Zdilla, Matthew. "The Pudendum and the Perversion of Anatomical Terminology." *Clinical Anatomy* 34, no. 5 (2021): 721–25.

Index

Note that italicized page numbers in this index indicate illustrative material.